Carol Sinclair was bor_____England in 1979. Married twice with one daughter and _____dren, she lives in Wiltshire and Wellington. A writer of both fact and fiction, she has always believed that fact is stranger than fiction. The story of how she learned that her low-starch diet for IBS was, in fact, treating an arthritic condition she didn't even know she had is an example. She worked in advertising, radio and television before becoming an author, and has published two adult novels, a biography of her husband Ray Harris Ching and a children's novel.

Visit Carol's website for further information: www.lowstarchdiet.net

The IBS
Low-Starch Diet

Carol Sinclair

Vermilion
LONDON

For Ray, my long-suffering husband whose tolerance for words such as starch,
ankylosing spondylitis, klebsiella and HLA-B27 has been severely tested in recent years,
but who has, nevertheless, listened patiently, worried endlessly about what is safe
for me to eat, and helped me through the bad times when I've eaten starch.

5 7 9 10 8 6

Published in the UK in 2003 by Vermilion, an imprint of Ebury Publishing
This revised edition published by Vermilion in 2006

Ebury Publishing is a Random House Group company

The Random House Group Limited Reg. No. 954009

Addresses for companies within the Random House Group can be found at
www.rbooks.co.uk

A CIP catalogue record for this book is available from the British Library

The Random House Group Limited supports The Forest Stewardship
Council (FSC), the leading international forest certification organisation.
All our titles that are printed on Greenpeace approved FSC certified paper
carry the FSC logo. Our paper procurement policy can be found at
www.rbooks.co.uk/environment

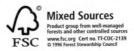

Mixed Sources
Product group from well-managed
forests and other controlled sources
www.fsc.org Cert no. TT-COC-2139
© 1996 Forest Stewardship Council
FSC

Printed in the UK by CPI Mackays, Chatham, ME5 8TD

ISBN 9780091912864

Copies are available at special rates for bulk orders. Contact the sales development
team on 020 7840 8487 or visit www.booksforpromotions.co.uk
for more information.

To buy books by your favourite authors and register for offers,
visit www.rbooks.co.uk

The advice offered in this book is not intended to be a substitute for the advice and
counsel of your personal physician. Always consult a medical practitioner before
embarking on a diet. Neither the author nor the publisher can be held responsible for
any loss or claim arising out of the use, or misuse, of the suggestions made, or the
failure to take medical advice.

WHAT IS STARCH?

Starch comes from plants – almost all foods made from *grains*: wheat, oats, rye, barley, corn, maize and rice; some *root vegetables*: potatoes, parsnips; some *green vegetables*: cabbage; and some *fruits*: bananas.

Starch is in all breakfast cereals, breads, cakes, pastries, pasta, batter, gravy and sauces made with flour, and most popular 'white foods' that often make you feel bloated and give you gut pain.

However, some grain products, such as alcohol and glucose syrup, are broken down into simple sugars during the processing and are *not* starch (see Chapter 6).

All starch is carbohydrate – but not all carbohydrate is starch

There are plant foods that don't contain starch, and ways of eating plant food so that the starch is not released into our digestive system.

Starch is made up of sugars

We know that too much sugar is bad for us. Sugars (the scientific name is *saccharides*) are the building blocks of starch. When you eat carbohydrates, your body doesn't ask: Is this honey? Is this sugar? Is this wheat flour? It only recognises them all as saccharides. Ordinary table sugar contains only two molecules of saccharide. Starch contains many hundreds, perhaps thousands, of saccharides. There's more 'sugar' in your bread than in your sugar bowl.

Starch is being added to our food in ever increasing ways

We're eating more starch than ever before. Look at the list of ingredients on food labels – you'll see that 'modified starch' is now added to most processed and prepared foods.

How to test for starch in your food

Iodine, when dropped onto food, goes very dark blue/black if the food contains starch. Get yourself a small bottle of iodine and an eye-dropper and you will always be able to tell which foods contain starch.

Starch causes digestive and arthritic problems for many people – but not for everyone

Many people can eat starch without health problems. Some people can eat *some* starch. This book will help you identify the symptoms caused by starch, and tell you how to find out which level of starch you can live with, and how to substitute starch in your food in many delicious ways.

CONTENTS

ACKNOWLEDGEMENTS

I would like to thank the following people: Alan Ebringer, Professor of Immunology, Division of Life Sciences, Infection and Immunity Group, King's College, London, for his great, inspirational discovery of how to treat AS by diet, his painstaking research and his kindness and concern for his patients.

My agent John McEwen, for his faith in the book and his untiring efforts on its behalf.

My editor Julia Kellaway, for her serene patience. Chris Benge of Kapiti Print Media Ltd, for his meticulous attention to detail and for cheerfully going the extra mile to get this edition right.

George McCaffery, for contacting me in 1999 to tell me that *The IBS Low-Starch Diet* also worked for AS, a disease I didn't even know I had.

Jane Barefoot, Senior Physiotherapist at the Royal National Hospital for Rheumatic Diseases, Bath, for personally guiding my description of AS symptoms and giving me her invaluable hands-on knowledge and experience of patients.

I am also indebted to: Andrei Calin, Consultant Rheumatologist, Royal National Hospital for Rheumatic Diseases, Bath, and Joel D. Taurog, Professor of Internal Medicine, Harold C. Simmons Arthritis Research Center, University of Texas Southwestern Medical Center, Dallas, USA, for their book *The Spondylarthritides*, which, with their many contributors, has given me so much information about the symptoms of AS.

Professor Muhammad Asim Khan, School of Medicine, Cleveland, USA, whose book *Ankylosing Spondylitis, the facts*, has also contributed to my knowledge of AS.

Fergus J. Rogers, Director of the National Ankylosing Spondylitis Society (NASS) London, and President of the Ankylosing Spondylitis International Federation (ASIF), for giving such insight into the AS patient's point of view.

The many IBS and AS sufferers who have written, phoned, faxed and e-mailed me with their questions and information.

PREFACE

How I found out that my IBS was really arthritis

This book is the culmination of a journey to find out what was causing my dreadful symptoms of gut pain and bloating diagnosed as irritable bowel syndrome (IBS) – and how they could be cured. It is also the story of an amazing discovery: the story of how – after I had found out how to end my symptoms, and after I had written a couple of books to help other people with IBS – I then discovered that my IBS is a symptom of an arthritic disease called ankylosing spondylitis, or AS.

I have written this book in the hope that it may provide a solution to the mystery of your chronic symptoms of pain and inflammation. On my journey I consulted many doctors, specialists and alternative medical practitioners. I read endless books on digestive problems. But no doctor or book was able to tell me why I was suffering from IBS, or what caused it.

When I discovered that the gut pain and bloating disappeared when I gave up eating starch, I knew I had at last found the solution to my agony. But it took many years of poring over textbooks, learning about starch, testing my theory and refining my diet until I could be absolutely sure.

Then in April 1999 George McCaffery, a patient of Alan Ebringer, Professor of Immunology at King's College, London, faxed me from Texas to say that he had discovered one of my books, *The IBS Starch-Free Diet*, on the Internet. George told me that he had AS, a painful, debilitating form of arthritis triggered by a microbe called *klebsiella*, which resides in the gut and lives on undigested starch. Professor Ebringer had been treating him with a low-starch diet and his symptoms had dramatically improved. He said that as far as he could see my book was the only starch diet book in the world, and he was sending a copy to Professor Ebringer.

From his description of the symptoms of AS – IBS is one of them – I began to wonder if perhaps I had been suffering from AS all along. A key to diagnosis is the HLA-B27 gene. Professor Ebringer advised me to have a blood test to see whether I have this gene. My GP agreed, and to my amazement I discovered that I am HLA-B27 positive. A further examination by Professor Ebringer, including an assessment of my medical history, confirmed that I do indeed have AS. Or rather, that I am in a pre-AS condition: my diet has prevented the visible symptoms.

I began to put the pieces of the puzzle together. Along with my gut pain and bloating I had years ago suffered from back pain, especially in the mornings before I got out of bed. I had consulted a specialist for jaw pain and clicking that made eating an agony. I had been treated with cortisone injections for severe shoulder pain – so bad that I had problems simply getting dressed. I had also had cortisone injections for pains in my elbows and arms which were so severe that I couldn't even lift a pot from the cupboard. And I'd gone to physiotherapists for my excruciating neck pains and stiffness. But I'd largely forgotten about all these, because some time ago they had faded away.

The more I thought about it, the more I realised that they had all disappeared at about the time I began eliminating starch from my diet.

Diagnosis of AS is made many years after the disease strikes – and only when bone degeneration can be seen on X-rays. People with the disease suffer for many years with pain and inflammation all over the body before being diagnosed. Even then there is no cure. I cannot be diagnosed as having AS on the evidence of skeletal X-rays because I have no visible signs of arthritis, no crippling or spinal degeneration. But I've now learned a lot about the disease, and recognise that I have had classic symptoms of pain and stiffness all over my body, from my jaw to my feet. Although I consulted doctors and specialists for each of these symptoms time and time again, the possibility of AS was never mentioned. But I now know that I would probably be in a wheelchair today if I hadn't discovered the IBS Low-Starch Diet.

When I consulted Professor Ebringer with my medical history he also asked me about my family history, because AS is a genetic disease and is passed down in families. Although I was born in New Zealand, my forebears all originate from areas of the world that have very high rates of the HLA-B27 gene: Sweden, Denmark, Shetland and Scotland. Many members of my family suffer from the same symptoms; some have now been diagnosed with AS.

AS causes inflammation all over the body – including in the gut. This is why IBS can be a symptom of AS. Some people suffer more severely from the gut pain and bloating, some from the arthritic symptoms. When I began my diet IBS was my most agonising symptom: the remission of back and joint pains was a bonus. For others, like George, the arthritic pain and crippling has always been the worst symptom.

If you are suffering from IBS, you may in fact have AS. Even if the cause of your IBS is not AS, the diet will work for you. But there are many undiagnosed or misdiagnosed sufferers out there. This book will tell you all you need to know to get a proper diagnosis, give you a long-term system for eating that will eliminate your symptoms – and transform your life.

Carol Sinclair, 2006

FOREWORD

Dr Alan Ebringer, B.Sc, MD, FRCP, FRACP, FRCPath, Professor of Immunology, King's College, University of London, Hon. Consultant in Rheumatology, UCL School of Medicine, Middlesex Hospital, London, and Consultant on Autoimmune Diseases to the National Institute of Health, Washington.

This excellent book by Carol Sinclair on the use of a 'low-starch diet' in people who suffer from backache and ankylosing spondylitis provides a long-awaited answer to repeated questions asked by patients who suffer from these all-too-common disorders.

Many patients receive a plentiful supply of drugs that may reduce their symptoms but they always ask: 'Doctor, what can I do to help myself? Could a diet help me?'

Carol Sinclair's book provides a clear and explicit answer to these questions as well as a simple and practical dietary method by which the patients can help themselves.

Ankylosing spondylitis is an arthritis involving the spine and large joints. The main symptoms are backache, usually in the lumbar area, which is worse in the mornings on getting up. Lumbar backache is often associated with muscle stiffness, so much so that the patient cannot get out of bed or does so with great difficulty. A characteristic, almost diagnostic, feature of this condition is that the muscle stiffness can be relieved by exercise.

There are approximately one million individuals in the UK and over five million in the United States who suffer from ankylosing spondylitis or from the early stages of this disease. It usually starts in the teens or twenties and affects men more frequently than women.

However, one of the greatest problems in ankylosing spondylitis is that it takes five to ten years or even twenty years to make a diagnosis, during which time the patient suffers from recurrent episodes of backache and muscle stiffness but is often accused of being neurotic or even malingering.

The main reason for 'delay to diagnosis' is that one of the definitions for this disease is 'presence of sacro-iliitis' on X-ray examination of the sacro-iliac joints. However, it takes five to ten years or even twenty years to develop sacro-iliitis which can be seen on radiological examination. Therefore the patients are told: 'You cannot have ankylosing spondylitis because you do not have sacro-iliitis.'

Nothing upsets patients more than to be told: 'There is nothing wrong with you, it is muscle strain, lumbago, stress, nerves or you are just imagining it.' However, a diet might resolve these problems and this book by Carol Sinclair could show how to achieve a possible reduction in symptoms.

A breakthrough in the study of ankylosing spondylitis occurred some thirty years ago, in 1973, when two groups of research workers, one from London and the other from Los Angeles, showed that over 95 per cent of patients with ankylosing spondylitis possess a particular white cell blood group, called 'human leucocyte antigen B-27', or HLA-B27 for short, but this blood group occurs in only 8 per cent of the general population.

This remarkable observation indicated that ankylosing spondylitis is almost completely confined to people who have this genetic blood group which they inherited from their parents. It had been known for almost a century that ankylosing spondylitis appeared to run in families but, up to 1973, it was not known which gene was responsible for this association. The discovery that almost all patients suffering from ankylosing spondylitis have the HLA-B27 blood group suggested that this marker was somehow involved with this disease. The presence of the HLA-B27 marker could be used to diagnose early cases of ankylosing spondylitis.

However, not all individuals who possess the HLA-B27 blood group will develop ankylosing spondylitis. Only 10 to 20 per cent of individuals who are HLA-B27 positive have some symptoms of ankylosing spondylitis, such as lumbar backache or muscle stiffness or both. Therefore it strongly suggests that for an individual to develop this condition, there must be present an environmental factor which, together with the genetic blood group HLA-B27, will trigger the onset of the disease.

The important scientific question arises: 'What is the nature of this environmental factor which can trigger backache in an individual who has been born with the blood group HLA-B27?' In 1975, our group at King's College and the Middlesex Hospital in London decided to study this and try to find the trigger factor with the question: 'Could an environmental agent be identified in patients with this disease and at the same time explain why it was linked to HLA-B27?'

The theoretical model used to investigate this problem was provided by the disease rheumatic fever. This condition, which affects the heart, is caused by antibodies produced by the patient himself or herself when they have an upper respiratory tract infection, a sore throat or tonsillitis due to streptococcus microbes. The streptococcus microbes have molecules that resemble those of the human heart. So, when tonsils are infected by streptococcus microbes, the immune system of the patient produces antibodies which attack both the microbes themselves and the body's own tissues, such as the heart, because of this shared molecular similarity or molecular mimicry.

When a disease occurs which is produced by the immune system of the patient, by its own antibodies, which are known as autoantibodies, such a condition is called an 'autoimmune disease'. Rheumatic fever is an autoimmune disease evoked by streptococcus microbes which carry molecules resembling the human heart. The rheumatic fever model suggested the hypothesis that ankylosing spondylitis patients had been infected by a microbe that possessed molecules resembling the blood group HLA-B27 and that it was therefore also an autoimmune disease.

This provided a possible explanation as to why the majority of ankylosing spondylitis patients belonged to the HLA-B27 blood group. Since only 10 or 20 per cent of HLA-B27 positive individuals had been exposed to this microbe, they, and only they, went on to develop the disease. This explained why the majority of individuals who were HLA-B27 positive, but who had not been exposed to this environmental factor, remained healthy and free from backache.

To identify this microbe, rabbits were injected with human HLA-B27 positive lymphocytes and the resultant serum tested against a number of different microorganisms. The environmental agent that was identified by the King's College/Middlesex Hospital group was a bowel microbe called *klebsiella*. The *klebsiella* microbes appeared to have molecules that resembled the HLA-B27 blood group and also the collagens found in the spine and the large joints. *Klebsiella* microbes are a normal component of the human bowel flora but ankylosing spondylitis patients were found to have greater quantities of this microbe in their stools when faecal specimens were examined using microbiological methods.

Furthermore, elevated levels of antibodies to *klebsiella* microbes were found in the blood of ankylosing spondylitis patients attending the Middlesex Hospital in London. These antibodies were easily detected, especially during the active phases of the disease when the patients had inflammatory flare-ups and severe episodes of backache. The London results were subsequently confirmed when similar observations were obtained by research groups from other clinical centres.

Elevated levels of antibodies against *klebsiella* microbes in ankylosing spondylitis patients have now been reported from the following countries: England, Scotland, USA, Finland, Slovakia, Canada, China, Germany, Spain, Turkey, Japan, Mexico, Netherlands, Taiwan, Australia and India. Clearly *klebsiella* microbes appear to be involved in ankylosing spondylitis patients throughout the world, irrespective of race or culture, but in all these countries the majority of patients still belong to the HLA-B27 positive genetic group.

Several nutritional studies have demonstrated that the main substrate for bacterial growth in the colon comes from dietary starch.

Therefore, a simple method of reducing the *klebsiella* bowel flora would be to lower the intake of dietary starch, to ask the patients to eat less-starchy foods. The 'London AS Diet' consists of a drastic reduction in starch consumption and to compensate for the calorie loss, the patients were asked to increase their intake of vegetables and proteins. The main principle or mantra of the 'London AS Diet' is: NO BREAD, NO POTATOES, NO CAKES and NO PASTA.

Some 400 ankylosing spondylitis patients have been treated over the last twenty years in the 'Ankylosing Spondylitis Research Clinic' of the Middlesex Hospital in London with this 'Low-Starch Diet'. The diet was used together with the usual drugs prescribed for ankylosing spondylitis such as sulphasalazine and indomethacin. Many of the non-steroidal anti-inflammatory drugs produce serious side-effects such as gastritis and gastro-intestinal bleeding. However, it was found that, used together with the 'London AS Low-Starch Diet', therapeutic effectiveness could be achieved with much lower doses of drugs, which thereby provided an added advantage to the patients being treated by both diet and various pharmaceutical preparations.

The low-starch diet is especially effective in the early stages of the disease, before severe bony changes have developed in the spine and caused irreversible damage. This lucid book by Carol Sinclair provides a more detailed description of the low-starch diet and allows the patient who is HLA-B27 positive to actively participate in the treatment of his or her disease. The great advantage of such a book is that the patient remains in control of dietary intake and can assess for himself or herself which dietary component is best suited for his or her condition.

The clear hope and intention is that this book will help you, if you are HLA-B27 positive, to achieve some relief from your painful symptoms. It is important to know whether you are HLA-B27 positive or not, because the diet is not so effective in individuals who do not possess this blood group. The test needs to be done only once in your life and your doctor will help you to obtain this information.

Although some patients obtain significant reduction in their symptoms, you should continue with your usual medication and your doctor should be informed of your dietary changes.

Not all patients respond to the low-starch diet; many are quite fond of their bread, potatoes or pasta. However, until you have tried the diet, you will not know whether it is good for you or not. This book will allow you to answer this question for yourself.

Your backache is an important problem for you and it is time you should become involved in its treatment.

1

What is IBS?

So. You've been diagnosed with IBS. You've been told it's due to stress – it's all in the mind – and been given tablets to reduce the pain. You've tried all sorts of remedies: herbal treatments, alternative medicine, tranquillisers, advice from friends, but nothing has worked.

And now, although you can see why the doctor says it's due to stress (because the more IBS you have, the more stressed you get), you begin to think, 'But lots of people have stress. Some lead far more stressful lives than I do. If it's due to stress, why doesn't everyone have it?'

There may be a number of types of IBS caused by different conditions. Doctors have various opinions and try various treatments. But there is one type of IBS which *can* be controlled by the IBS Low-Starch Diet. It has nothing to do with stressful living. It is *physiological* (caused by your body) and not *psychological* ('all in the mind').

What are the symptoms?

The symptoms begin with a feeling of fullness or bloating in the gut (you may think of it as your stomach) usually quite soon after a meal. This can happen after any meal, but in my experience it is more usual after the evening meal.

The bloating may begin during the meal (depends how long you linger at the table) and will increase until you feel the need to loosen your belt. It will then become a disquieting ache, turning into small, nagging jabs of pain, and within several hours it will become waves of agony surging through your distended stomach – sometimes worse than labour pains.

At this stage you will long to lie down. Sometimes you'll be at a dinner party and will have to keep smiling and enduring the pain. But if you're at home, you will, no doubt, go to bed. I've been in such pain at this stage that I couldn't walk up the stairs – I've had to crawl.

Throughout the night the pain will continue in waves, moving from the right side of your abdomen to the left, and then lower down. Some people may also vomit at this stage. When the pain gets lower you will perhaps be able to pass a bowel motion. Some people will have diarrhoea; some (like me) will be constipated. Both conditions are associated with IBS.

Usually by morning the pain has receded, although you may still have a feeling of bloatedness, which will be with you during the day and will slowly increase until your evening meal, at which stage the whole cycle will begin again. In my experience, this cycle sometimes goes on for about three days before subsiding.

Sometimes, however, the pain can be so severe that you may be admitted to hospital with volvulus. This is a twisting of part of the bowel caused by the build-up of gas in your intestine. It may untwist spontaneously or by manipulation, but surgical exploration is often performed.

When you are younger you may experience IBS less severely and only occasionally – but enough to recognise the signs and learn to dread them. As you get older, it will usually become more frequent. In my case I can remember experiencing the pain and bloating as a child. But it wasn't until my teenage years that it began to affect me badly. By middle age it was a permanent and desperate part of my life, occurring almost every night.

By this time I had been diagnosed as having IBS, but no doctor could give me a satisfactory explanation of what caused it. I was always told only that it was due to stress. This, of course, made me feel that it was all my fault.

What does IBS actually mean?

The term 'IBS' has become so well known that we tend to gloss over what it actually is. It is in fact a vague description for what may be a range of symptoms. The words 'irritable bowel syndrome' have no specific medical meaning. They mean just what they say: your bowel becomes (for some unknown reason) irritable – or upset. Why this irritation comes about, or what causes it, is not understood.

But one thing doctors do know, and despair of, is that IBS is increasing in both Western and Oriental populations. Indeed, it has become so common that it could be called an epidemic. It is estimated that between 14 and 22 per cent of the general population suffer the symptoms at some time in their life. Two-thirds of IBS sufferers are women. The onset of symptoms occurs before the age of thirty-five years in 50 per cent of patients. For men it is often younger, at around the age of twenty. Constipation is more common in women and diarrhoea more common in men.

If doctors don't know what causes IBS, how do they diagnose it?

In 1992, a group of bowel experts met in Rome and described the main symptoms of IBS. They agreed that if a patient had some or all of these symptoms for at least three months, and if they recurred, the patient could be said to be suffering from IBS. The symptoms include abdominal discomfort or pain which is:

- relieved by defecation (a bowel motion); and/or
- associated with a change in how often you have a bowel motion; and/or
- associated with a change in the consistency of your stool (faeces becoming harder or softer).

In addition, if there are two or more of the following symptoms at least 25 per cent of the time, the diagnosis will be confirmed as IBS:

- abdominal bloating and distension;
- more than three stools a day or less than three a week;
- erratic and/or unsatisfactory bowel motions (straining, urgency or a feeling of incomplete evacuation);
- mucus or slime in the stool;
- nausea or loss of appetite.

Some IBS-like symptoms are signs of other bowel diseases

There are other, more serious bowel conditions, such as Crohn's disease or ulcerative colitis, which may also include symptoms similar to IBS. You should be sure to tell your doctor if you have experienced very dramatic abdominal pain coupled with loss of weight, pain or difficulty in swallowing food, any blood in your stools or if they are very dark in colour, or if you have had any fever.

If you have recently had an abdominal operation, if a near relative, such as mother, father, sister or brother, has developed bowel cancer under the age of fifty years, or if, as a woman, you have any vaginal discharge, period problems or pain on intercourse, you should also be sure to inform your doctor. He may need to arrange for you to see a hospital specialist.

Diverticulosis is another bowel condition which will give similar symptoms. This is when weaknesses develop in the wall of the bowel, forming small pouches or diverticulae. Partly digested food can become trapped in these pouches, causing putrefaction and a build-up of gas. Diverticulosis usually develops as one gets older and it is perfectly possible to have this condition as well as, or as a result of, IBS, because it is usually caused by years of constipation.

My search for the cause of my IBS

Diagnosis of my IBS was made long before the experts in Rome had drawn up that list of symptoms. On the basis of that list I might not have been diagnosed as having IBS.

My abdominal discomfort or pain could not usually be relieved by defecation – because I was always constipated and had particular trouble defecating when I was having an IBS attack.

I could not say that the IBS pain was associated with a change in how *often* I had a bowel motion – because for as long as I could remember my bowel motions had been few and far between. Sometimes I would go as long as four weeks without a bowel motion.

Also, the IBS pain was not due to a change in the consistency of my stool – it had always been as hard as a rock.

Although my constipation was miserable and uncomfortable, it didn't necessarily mean I had pain and bloating. I could never work out why or when I would get IBS symptoms, or what had caused them.

I tried anything and everything

When I first began going to doctors to find out why I had pain and bloating, I was told I had spastic bowel, which was caused by stress. I went through a series of barium X-rays and was told that I had a megacolon (long, narrow colon) with weak muscle tone. The only advice I was given was to 'keep regular', so I began taking laxatives.

The laxatives made me feel sick, but did increase my number of bowel motions. However, they made no difference at all to the pain and bloating.

Then the new phrase, irritable bowel syndrome, began to be used and I was diagnosed with IBS. This made no difference to the advice I was given about my condition, which was still thought to be due to stress, but I was told that eating more roughage would help.

My mother had always believed in healthy eating and I'd been eating brown bread and bran muffins from childhood, but now I began to redouble my efforts. Muesli, bran and wholemeal bread were part of almost every meal. Not only did it make no difference to the pain and bloating, but I began to get more constipated, so I increased my intake of laxatives.

I then heard that yoghurt was good for the bowel, so I began each day with a carton of yoghurt mixed with bran. It made no difference to the IBS and I continued to get more constipated. So once again I increased my intake of laxatives.

Finally I began taking various herbal pills and remedies, trying all sorts of alternative medicine, but the relentless increase in both my constipation and my IBS never stopped.

I was told I had an IBS personality. Of course I did! I was often depressed, anxious, hostile, miserable and fatigued. Anyone suffering constant mysterious, undiagnosed pain goes through these moods. Sometimes I used to think I *was* a hypochondriac, neurotically producing symptoms of all sorts of illnesses, even convinced I had undiagnosed gall bladder and bowel cancer. I can remember going to bed and crying with weakness and pain, feeling black moods of despair and anger.

IBS is a complex problem. There may be a number of causes. But it's all too easy to convince sufferers that it's all in the mind. Almost everyone experiences stress or emotional problems of some kind, so it's very convenient for doctors to be able to diagnose 'stress' as the cause of a patient's symptoms – no one can argue with it. It's also guaranteed to increase stress by making many patients – particularly women – feel guilty about their inability to manage their relationships/job/children. The vicious circle can escalate as some patients attempt to blame their family or employers for their stress. Some of us slink away timidly, ashamed of bothering the doctor, vowing to try harder to overcome our stress. Others opt for tranquillisers or a course of counselling. But none of these options will help the patient to overcome IBS. Stress is the worst and most unhelpful diagnosis a doctor can give.

I began to get lucky

In 1986, when I was at my wits' end, I was lucky enough to tune into a TV documentary about Dr John Hunter's work on food allergies, which claimed that eliminating wheat from the diet could successfully eliminate IBS symptoms. I immediately gave up everything made from wheat flour, wholegrains or wheat bran, and experienced a dramatic decrease in pain and bloating. However, about eighteen months later the symptoms began to return sporadically.

In 1987 I was admitted to St Mark's Hospital in London for

gastrointestinal tests to see whether perhaps I had a condition called Hirschprung's disease, which is paralysis of part of the bowel. I was sure the surgeons would operate to remove the offending part and that I would live happily ever after.

It was a terrible disappointment to be told that they couldn't be sure I had Hirschprung's disease, and in any case an operation would not necessarily be successful – and even if it was, it wouldn't change my symptoms of pain and bloating. I have since been enormously grateful to the surgeons at St Mark's for not operating. It would only have compounded my problems.

One fortunate aspect of that hospital stay was that I was advised to give up laxatives (by that time I was taking thirty-five Senokot a night) and switch to Epsom salts. I didn't realise it, but I had become addicted to laxatives. Addiction is when you have to keep increasing the dose to get the same results. Epsom salts, on the other hand, is a non-addictive, natural laxative that has many other benefits. There is more about this in Chapter 11, 'What can I eat?', with an explanation of why your doctor won't have told you about it.

So St Mark's couldn't cure my IBS, but the advice about Epsom salts alone was worth the two uncomfortable weeks I spent there, going through a most horrible range of tests.

From medical mouse to laboratory rat

I left St Mark's determined to find out what other foods, in addition to wheat, were causing my pain and bloating. I finally discovered it was starch, but this took many years and much testing. Being your own laboratory rat is no fun, but the remission of symptoms was so wonderful that it made me very determined to find out exactly what starch was, and why it was causing me such pain.

Although IBS is always considered to be connected with either constipation or diarrhoea, I've discovered that the pain and bloating can be separately controlled. A few years ago, while I was undergoing a series of X-rays to confirm my megacolon diagnosis, I was not allowed to take Epsom salts or other laxatives for ten days. During that time I stuck to my low-starch diet, and although I was constipated the whole time, I had no IBS pain or even bloating.

The final pieces of the puzzle only fell into place in 1999, when I discovered the real cause of my IBS. By that time I had found a way to eliminate the symptoms and had written a book about it. But it took an extraordinary and unexpected piece of information from a stranger to reveal the actual nature of my IBS.

My type of IBS is one of a group of inflammatory diseases which includes a form of arthritis, and which can be identified by a particular genetic marker. Many of the overlapping symptoms are not normally thought of as being all part of one disease. Most doctors treat these conditions separately, usually with anti-inflammatory drugs, and do not understand that they can be controlled by diet.

If you have the genetic marker, you are in the high-risk group and may develop any or some of these symptoms, including IBS. This book will tell you how to find out if your IBS is caused by this gene, and how to treat your symptoms.

Not everyone who has IBS falls into this genetic group. But many IBS sufferers, regardless of their genetic make-up, find that the IBS Low-Starch Diet eliminates their IBS symptoms.

I strongly believe that the cause of IBS is overwhelmingly physiological, not psychological

When I began my diet, most doctors believed IBS was all in the mind. And although there is still much emphasis on stress as being the underlying cause, some doctors are now beginning to believe that food intolerance is the major factor. However, most of the researchers in this field still don't know why.

Research in this area is very difficult. Studies have shown that cereals, especially wheat, and dairy foods are most to blame. But researchers have still not shown any understanding of the connection between these food groups and why such completely different foods should cause the same problem.

All these foods contain *starch* in some degree. In the case of dairy foods, it is not called starch – it is called lactose, one of the component sugars of starch. Since few understand that it is starch which is the culprit, or the difference between starch and carbohydrates, it is not surprising that present research produces unreliable results.

There are many hidden starches in our diet. Even medications usually contain starch in tiny amounts. But it is very easy to test for starch – even a child can do it. I have discovered how sensitive certain people (I am one) can be to the smallest amounts of starch. Without an understanding of this, researchers find that results vary between their studies.

Researchers also find it difficult to get people to stick to the diets they devise. Doctors know this, but feel the diets are unpalatable and that they are depriving their patients. They are also worried about the diets being nutritionally inadequate. Because they don't understand that it is starch they should be eliminating, they don't understand what is safe to eat, and the range of delicious, nutritious substitute foods that are available.

Not everyone who has IBS is as sensitive to starch as I am. You may not need to give up all the starchy foods I live happily without. But once you know it is starch that is causing your problems, you can decide what level of starch you can live with. You may only need to avoid starch on occasions when you want to look and feel your best – for that special dinner date or at a party, for example.

If my description of IBS sounds similar to your symptoms, you can begin the IBS Low-Starch Diet for yourself today. But to find out the actual nature of your IBS and whether you may be in the high-risk group for additional symptoms, get correctly diagnosed. This book will tell you how.

2

Ever been told the pain in your back is all in your mind?

I bet you have – because your backache and/or joint pain has probably been coming and going in a mysterious way for years. Sounds ridiculous when you explain it to the doctor, but sometimes it's in one part of your back, sometimes in another. Sometimes it's in your shoulders, neck or even your jaw. Perhaps you feel pain and stiffness in your back which seems to move around in a way that is difficult to describe. And you may have other symptoms which you don't think are related to the pain in your back. You may even be beginning to think of yourself as the hypochondriac other people believe you to be!

That's what happened to me for years and years, in my search for the cause of the pain in my gut. I went from doctor to doctor, desperate for a diagnosis of the awful symptoms of pain and bloating. The fact that I also had backache every morning – which got worse as I lay in bed until I was forced to get up – was, I thought, a separate problem. At various times I had suffered severe shoulder pains, arm and elbow pains, pain in my jaw, agonising neck pain and stiffness. I was told I had repetitive strain injury. I was prescribed cortisone injections for shoulder and elbow pain and referred to physiotherapists, all with varying degrees of relief for a while.

I also had mysterious symptoms which no one would explain: for about two years I suffered off and on from an excruciating form of cystitis in which I passed blood clots in my urine. I didn't know it at the time, but this can also be the symptom of a type of venereal disease. No doctor admitted as much to me, but they put me on a long course of very strong antibiotics, which ultimately cured this. So I thought these problems were under control, and I never connected them with my gut pain.

No doctor treating me for my joint pains ever told me I might have a type of arthritis. And when I went to the doctor about my gut pain, no one ever asked me if I also had backache or joint pains.

I went on for years, longing for a cure for the gut pain, even grateful in the end for the diagnosis of IBS, despite the doctors telling me it was due to stress – all in the mind.

I bought all the books on IBS, spent years trying alternative remedies, until I began to realise that the books were all copies of each other, and none of them helped me. And the alternative remedies either did not work or made me worse.

Then I was lucky enough to stumble on the idea of giving up starch – and I mean stumble! Even though my first efforts at giving up wheat flour were dramatically successful, it took me years to discover that the real problem was starch and how to live without it.

But it was still some years until I made the amazing discovery that gut pain, backache, joint pains and the other symptoms I had are often (not always) one and the same arthritic disease. It is a real disease – it's not all in your mind, and it's not due to stress.

At this point I must clarify which type of stress I'm talking about. Most people – even doctors – use the word 'stress' to describe our emotional or mental reactions to the problems of life. Relationships breaking up. Working too hard. Death of a loved one. Money worries. This type of stress I do not believe will cause the symptoms of gut pain or backache.

However, the physical stress your body may suffer from an accident or illness can cause these symptoms. It is known that accidents which cause damage to bones and joints can trigger arthritic problems. There are also accounts of episodes and/or epidemics such as dysentery causing sufferers to develop arthritis. For those of us with a genetic disposition, this type of stress can cause our immune systems to malfunction, and this can be the key to the emergence of gut pain and backache.

But if, as a result of physical stress, you begin to show symptoms of gut and joint pains and these are not correctly diagnosed, you will also begin to show symptoms of emotional stress. I've been told that I had a 'low pain threshold', or that my symptoms were due to psychological factors – even that I had an IBS personality. Of course I did! Not only was I experiencing constant pain which no one could cure, but they kept telling me I was neurotic. Enough to make anyone emotionally stressed.

If you have suffered from chronic gut pain, backache and joint pain for a number of years; if there have been similar symptoms in your family; if you have seen many specialists, had investigations and treatments, tried alternative medicine and been to a number of therapists; if everyone has given you a different diagnosis and no one has been able to give you lasting relief, you are probably suffering from a type of inflammatory arthritis which has not yet been diagnosed because the symptoms usually become recognisable only in later life – when it's too late.

Just as IBS sufferers are often told it is all in the mind, many sufferers of chronic backache are considered neurotic. You may even have been referred to a psychiatrist for counselling. Your family and friends will probably have lost patience with you and you may be feeling very frustrated, angry and alone. You know the pain is real – but to other people you are just a malingerer.

Finally you have come to the conclusion that your doctor cannot do anything more than tell you to stay on the pain-relieving drugs, avoid lifting, get lots of bed rest, try heat massage or localised creams or sprays, and exercise.

If this has been the history of your backache and joint pain – if you've been told that your gut pain is due to stress – there is still something you can do.

Get correctly diagnosed – the answer is in your genes

The first thing to do is to find out whether your type of backache, joint pain and gut pain can be controlled by diet. Ask your GP to arrange for a blood test to discover whether you have the HLA-B27 gene. If a blood test reveals that you have this gene, you are in the high-risk group for ankylosing spondylitis, or AS.

What is ankylosing spondylitis?

Although you may never have heard of it before, AS is as common as rheumatoid arthritis and far more common than better-known diseases such as leukaemia, muscular dystrophy and cystic fibrosis.

AS is a chronic (in other words, it doesn't go away) inflammatory form of arthritis which runs in families. Other names for it include poker back or bamboo spine. These old-fashioned names refer to the rigidity which develops if the spine is badly affected.

AS is one of a group of diseases which includes Reiter's syndrome, psoriatic arthritis, colitic arthritis and inflammatory bowel diseases (which in the early years may be diagnosed as IBS). Many of the overlapping symptoms are not normally thought of as being arthritic.

Approximately one in 200 adults in the UK has been diagnosed with AS and if you consider that one in five adults in the UK has been diagnosed with IBS – and that they may in fact have AS – it will give you an idea of the numbers of people suffering from this disease.

What's the difference between rheumatism and arthritis?

There are over 200 different types of rheumatic disease, some of which are extremely unusual. Rheumatism is a general term for any disorder in which aches and pains affect the muscles and joints. A rheumatologist treats both rheumatism and arthritis. The general term 'rheumatism' may be used to describe aches and pains which can affect bones, muscles and ligaments unrelated to arthritis – if, for example, you strain a muscle.

Just as the names tonsill*itis* and appendic*itis* are used for disease and inflammation in other parts of the body ('itis' always means inflammation), arthr*itis* is the general term for disease and inflammation which causes damage to a joint. But it is also used to describe any sort of joint disease, even when there is no inflammation involved. There are many types of arthritis and many causes.

What are the symptoms of AS?

AS can affect your eyes, jaw, neck, shoulders, breastbone, rib joints, spine, bowels, sacroiliac joints, hips, knees, ankles, heels, Achilles tendon and the joints of the foot – in other words, many parts of the body. However, for years before the disease is diagnosed, some people with AS suffer primarily from backache and/or gut pain and bloating.

Gut pain and bloating

May come and go. You will notice it is worse after meals, especially in the evening. You will usually feel better in the morning. It will get more frequent as you get older. You may be told that it is colitis or spastic bowel or IBS or IBD (inflammatory bowel disease) or nonspecific gut inflammation. In extreme cases it can result in intestinal obstruction and volvulus (a twisting or kinking of the small bowel). You may be rushed to hospital. Emergency surgery may have to be performed. Many people with Crohn's disease or ulcerative colitis may also develop AS.

Backache

Begins insidiously over a period of weeks, usually with pain and stiffness in the lower back which comes and goes, and can move to different areas of the spine. This may cause pain down the front or the back of one thigh, then the other, as the inflammation presses on the sciatic nerve. This may be diagnosed simply as sciatica. For many years you may have experienced disturbed sleep. Sleeping on your side may cause pain in your shoulders and neck. You may experience tension in your neck and feel you are unable to completely relax. You may spend much of the night rearranging your pillows, trying to get a more comfortable position. Back pain may be worse in the small hours, finally forcing you out of bed. And when you do get up, you'll feel stiff. This is always worse in the mornings. Turning the head, bending or stooping may be difficult, if not impossible, without pain. You may believe you simply have a strained back. In the early stages the pain and stiffness will recede during the day. Eventually there will be longer periods of exacerbation and then remission of the inflammation and pain.

Shoulders, neck, hips, knees, ankles and arms

Can all be affected by pain and stiffness. Sometimes this is misdiagnosed as repetitive strain injury (RSI) and treated with cortisone injections, which can bring relief to the painful area.

Eye pain

This may have been diagnosed as iritis, and can be another serious symptom. You may experience pain in one eye, redness, blurred vision, a dislike of bright light. Inflammation can affect any portion of the eye or surrounding orbital tissue and cause various conditions from conjunctivitis to a serious one called acute anterior uveitis. This is treated quite differently from the other conditions and requires urgent diagnosis. For correct diagnosis of the seriousness of this condition, it is helpful to know whether you are HLA-B27 positive, as an ophthalmologist will then know what treatment to give. If you experience these symptoms and know you are HLA-B27 positive, you should go immediately to the eye section in the Accident and Emergency department of your local hospital and tell them you are HLA-B27 positive. Do not wait for a GP's referral.

Breathing difficulties

May make you feel as if your breathing is always too shallow and you can't fill your lungs with enough fresh air. Some people find it painful to breathe deeply. Sneezing, coughing or yawning can also be painful. This is due to the slow, subtle stiffening of your rib and sternum joints as the disease progresses. Pain in the ribs is a common feature of AS and may begin before you are aware of any chest restriction. You may fear that it is a heart condition. Breathing exercises and remembering to adopt a good posture will help.

Feet and heels

May sometimes ache. Pain can occur underneath the heel bone and/or underneath the foot about three centimetres from the back of the foot, and/or underneath the ball of the foot. The back of the heel, where the Achilles tendon is attached to the bone, may also be painful.

Skin rashes

These may have been diagnosed as psoriasis. You may notice that they become worse under sunlight or ultraviolet light. On the other hand, sometimes they improve with sunlight. Most commonly itchy, dry, red and scaly patches of skin will develop and, sometimes, finger and toenails may show discoloration and pitting. There are a number of forms of psoriasis, some quite mild and some very severe. In its most severe form it is an associated disease known as psoriatic arthritis.

Reiter's syndrome

Another associated condition, in the past considered to be primarily a disease of men. In addition to all the painful inflammatory symptoms described above, it causes symptoms resembling gonorrhoea and discharge from the penis. It is now known that women can also have this disease. This takes the form of acute haemorrhagic cystitis (extreme need to pass urine, along with bleeding or clots of blood in the urine) and is extremely painful, but the urethral symptoms can respond to long-term antibiotic therapy.

Childhood onset

AS can begin from the age of around ten years, with pain and tenderness in the knee, groin, hip, ankle or other large joints. This is often dismissed as 'growing pains'. The child may limp from time to time, without having an injury. If there is a family history of AS, psoriasis, inflammatory bowel disease or acute iritis, it should be investigated with a blood test. If the child is found to be HLA-B27 positive, adult AS symptoms will usually develop in later life.

The AS 'stigmata'

All these symptoms are known as the 'stigmata' or signs of the disease. You may have a number of them, or only one. You may have had many minor indications throughout your life, but have taken no notice of them, or shrugged them off with explanations passed down from older members of the family. If you complained of sore joints when you were a child, you were probably told they were 'growing pains'.

As you get older you may have woken up with a stiff neck or painful stiff back. When you've mentioned it, you may have been told it was because you've slept in a draught, or an uncomfortable position, with too many pillows, even that you have a 'cold in your back'.

You will probably hear many such explanations from family members, because there have probably been many such symptoms throughout your family. You may also have bowel problems, either constipation, which will have been treated with high-grain cereals or laxatives, or diarrhoea, which you will probably have been told is due to stress or a nervous disposition – as with your gut pain.

What causes the symptoms?

What is happening to you is that inflammation is beginning to spread throughout your body, although often the two major areas affected are your joints and your gut.

The term IBS is vague, and only refers to your symptoms of pain and bloating. However, inflammation is occurring in your gastrointestinal tract and can take various forms. If tests are done to find out what is causing this, your specialist may say you have IBD, or Crohn's disease, or ulcerative colitis.

In your joints and spine, inflammation is beginning at the edges of the bones and between the vertebrae. When the inflammation dies down, bone grows from both sides of the joint as part of a healing process. But eventually the bone can surround the joint completely, making it rigid.

Ultimately, in its most severe untreated form, AS may leave you with a hunchback and/or severe disability. But this does not always become obvious for many years. When you become aware of AS, you will see elderly people in the street, or the supermarket, with the hunched back of AS sufferers. This does not always cause severe pain, but sometimes it can result in the sufferer being unable to lift their head. But you will be glad to know that even without effective treatment, not everyone with AS has the most severe symptoms.

How is AS usually treated?

In the early stages you may be prescribed anti-inflammatory drugs, antibiotics or immunosuppressants. Some have dangerous side effects, both physical and psychological. Local cortisone injections may alleviate symptoms for a while. Surgery to fuse the spine is sometimes used in the United States as a last resort in extreme cases. This does not have a history of success. Some patients repeat this painful treatment several times, without permanent benefit. None of these treatments can do more than give temporary relief from pain. Conventional treatment is always palliative only and unsuccessful in halting the progress of the disease.

The worst problem of AS is misdiagnosis

Apart from the confusing range of overlapping symptoms, there are many myths and misconceptions about AS which make it difficult to get an early diagnosis. It has always been considered to be more common in men. Indeed, it is often seen in quite young men. However, it is now recognised that it is often missed in women, or misdiagnosed. It may be that men in the early stages suffer more from the back-ache and stiffness symptoms, while women may experience the inflammatory bowel conditions and symptoms in the peripheral joints (i.e. away from the centre – wrists, knees, feet, etc). Doctors can't decide which comes first – the bowel problems or the joint problems – but both can be primary symptoms of AS, and you may experience both, in addition to others.

It is my opinion that the reason doctors have been slow to draw the conclusion that the bowel, back and joint symptoms are part of the same disease is that men with advanced AS are usually referred to a rheumatologist or perhaps an orthopaedic consultant, while women with IBS are referred to a gastroenterologist (if they're lucky) – two different branches of medicine with probably very little contact who, until recently, didn't realise they were working on the same disease. No wonder they didn't get it together.

It wasn't until immunology, another branch of medicine involved in genetic research, began to show the connection with the HLA-B27 gene that these, and many other symptoms, were recognised as part of the same syndrome.

Spondylarthropathy is a term that refers to different forms of inflammatory disease involving spinal and other symptoms. In fact the cycle of AS symptoms is now beginning to be called 'the spondylarthropathies' or 'the spondylarthritides'.

Your GP may not have heard of this yet, but doctors are not researchers and understandably, considering their workload, take a long time to catch up on new research.

3

How do genes cause my gut pain and backache?

The HLA-B27 gene is found in roughly 8 per cent of the UK population; this means there are approximately five million people in the country with the gene. The prevalence of the HLA-B27 gene differs in different populations and ethnic groups, throughout the world. Sometimes you will hear it called a 'marker', which means it marks you out as being in the high-risk group for a certain medical condition.

Not everyone with the HLA-B27 gene falls prey to AS, but between 10 and 20 per cent of those people in the UK with the HLA-B27 marker do suffer from it.

But genes alone do not cause disease

It was always known that AS is a 'reactive' condition; that is, that the disease is triggered by something – it reacts to some environmental or biological trigger. But what it reacts to, no one knew.

Genetic scientists had discovered that many reactive conditions are autoimmune. This means that for some mysterious reason, the body's immune system reacts against itself. This is exactly the opposite of what the immune system is supposed to do. Our immune system is like a defensive army within our body, ready to do war with the bacteria and viruses that invade us to cause illness. We don't think of these invaders as other life forms, but in fact they are. Without our immune system we would be taken over by these 'body snatchers'. Our immune system is constantly on the look-out; it knows what all the destructive bacteria and viruses look like and has been trained to send out warriors (antibodies) to destroy these invaders as soon as they enter our bodies.

Unfortunately, sometimes the invaders can look the same as the body's own genes. When this happens, the body inadvertently begins to destroy its own cells.

When it was discovered that over 96 per cent of patients with AS also had the HLA-B27 gene, researchers had their first clue. And in 1975, when Professor Ebringer and his team found that these patients also

17

had antibodies to a common bacterium, *Klebsiella pneumoniae*, which mimics the HLA-B27 gene, they were well on the way to solving the puzzle. As the immune system attempted to destroy the *klebsiella*, it was also destroying the B27 cells of the body, causing the painful inflammatory progress of AS.

The discovery that AS is an autoimmune disease was a huge advance. But how to overcome it was still not understood. Professor Ebringer believed that if the bacterium could be destroyed long-term, the immune system would register that the invader had gone and would stop attacking the B27 genes. *Klebsiella pneumoniae*, as the name suggests, can also cause pneumonia, and has been known about for a long time. It can be subdued by drugs, of course. The drug most commonly prescribed to subdue this bacterium was, and still is, sulphasalazine. This is one of the disease-modifying anti-rheumatic drugs (DMARDs), sometimes also called slow-acting anti-rheumatic drugs, and is effective for many people. But it has unpleasant side-effects, and if you come into contact with *klebsiella* again (as you surely will) you will be reinfected – and you don't want to live on sulphasalazine for the rest of your life. Moreover, although sulphasalazine works short-term, it does not seem to prevent the return of IBS in patients with AS.

How, then, could the *klebsiella* be destroyed in a way that was sustainable and did no harm to the body? If one could destroy what the *klebsiella* lived on in the body, perhaps one could destroy the bacterium? But where in the body did the *klebsiella* live, and what did it live on? For many years Professor Ebringer and his team struggled with the dilemma, knowing that the solution was very close. Finally the breakthrough discovery came.

How can diet destroy bacteria?

As with all great discoveries, the breakthrough didn't exactly come in the laboratory. One of Professor Ebringer's patients asked him to devise a weight-loss diet that would really work. Always unconventional, the professor recommended that he eat as much steak and as many tomatoes as he wanted, and drink a bottle of red wine daily. His patient thought this a wonderful joke, and told all his friends what a great diet his doctor had advised – much to their envious amusement. But he stuck to the diet for a month, lost weight and felt fantastic. When he went back to Professor Ebringer, he was a happy man. 'Not only have I lost weight,' he said, 'but my joint and back pains have disappeared!'

For Professor Ebringer, the penny dropped. He knew that his diet was very low in starch. He knew that when eating a normal starchy diet, all humans have partially undigested starch remaining in the gut (colon). He came to the conclusion that *klebsiella* must live on the partially undigested starch in the gut – and that his low-starch diet must have starved them, or at least subdued them enough to make the immune system no longer see them as a threat. Further research in the laboratory revealed that the gut is indeed where the *klebsiella* live and grow on remnants of the starch in our diets.

Professor Ebringer began putting his AS patients on a low-starch diet, with great success. Patients reported amazing relief from symptoms. But a low-starch diet seems, at first, too appalling to contemplate. Giving up all bread, pastry, pasta, cakes, potatoes, rice and so on is not easy. What does one eat? Unless one has a good knowledge of cooking and nutrition, substitute foods can be a mystery. Hidden starches are also being added to our diet in ever-increasing amounts, in processed and prepared foods. Patients have found it difficult to stick to the diet, without help.

This book is a practical and comprehensive plan for managing the diet on a daily and long-term basis. Not everyone needs to give up all forms of starch – it depends on how severe your symptoms are. The book tells you how to begin slowly, giving up the most starchy foods first and then, if necessary, the next food group. It tells you how to identify starch in your food with the simple iodine test. It gives you many delicious, nutritious recipes. It tells you how to eat out in restaurants. It makes a starch-free diet not only possible, but enjoyable.

Postscript

Although over 96 per cent of AS sufferers have the HLA-B27 gene, it is now thought that other associated genes, called subtypes, are also involved. The more disease-predisposing genes you inherit, the more likely you are to suffer from AS symptoms. The highest rates of both the B27 gene and AS are to be found in northern European countries, beginning with the people living closest to the North Pole: the Haida Indians in British Columbia, who have a 50 per cent rate of B27, and Siberian Eskimos (Inuits), who have a 40 per cent rate. The rate is high in Scandinavian countries, especially Finland. Although I was born in New Zealand, my forebears all originate from northern areas of the world with very high rates of the HLA-B27 gene: Sweden, Denmark, Shetland and Scotland. I may have inherited many different copies of

B27, and perhaps other subtypes. Perhaps this is why I have had so many symptoms in various areas of my body.

Further information about this is available from literature cited in the references at the back of the book.

Crohn's disease and the IBS Low-Starch Diet

Crohn's disease is a chronic inflammatory bowel disease which can involve any part of the gastrointestinal system – from the mouth to the anus.

The symptoms include cramping abdominal pains, especially after eating. Sometimes the pain is in the right-hand side of the abdomen and might be diagnosed as appendicitis. Nausea and diarrhoea, fever, appetite and weight loss, a general ill feeling, abdominal tenderness, often with swelling that feels like a 'mass' in the stomach, and sometimes black, tarry stools (faeces) or blood in the stools are all part of Crohn's disease

Usually the symptoms begin when the sufferer is in his/her early twenties and may continue every few months for several years with periods of relapse and remission. Occasionally the symptoms may appear only once or twice, and the disease may then disappear.

No one knows what causes Crohn's disease but for a long time it has been thought that it could be an autoimmune disease similar to AS. Most people with the disease do not have the HLA-B27 marker, but those who do go on to develop AS. Also, people with AS often develop Crohn's disease. One similarity to AS is that people with Crohn's disease have been shown to have antibodies to the *klebsiella* bacterium.

The incidence of Crohn's disease has increased steadily in recent years since World War II, particularly in the industrialised parts of the world; it is rare in underdeveloped countries. Some doctors believe that its rise is connected with our Western diet of highly processed foods. They admit that the foods that seem to cause problems for people with Crohn's disease are the same as those that cause problems for people with IBS, which they say are wheat and dairy foods. However, their dietary recommendations do not show any under-standing of starch, or the part that the elimination of starch might play in the remission of symptoms. A number of diets have been tried, and although some seem more successful than others, no one is sure which is best.

Conventional treatment for people with Crohn's disease is still with drugs, particularly anti-inflammatory drugs including cortisones, which have unpleasant and even dangerous side effects.

Professor Ebringer believes that the low-starch diet would also work for people with Crohn's disease. If I had Crohn's disease, I would certainly try the IBS Low-Starch Diet.

Coeliac disease and the IBS Low-Starch Diet

Coeliac disease (spelt 'celiac' in the US and pronounced that way in the UK), thought for years to be quite rare, has recently been discovered to be a common, but badly understood, condition.

The classic symptoms, which until recently have been considered to be the only symptoms, are poor appetite, loose, pale, bulky, bad-smelling stools, frequent gas, swollen abdomen, abdominal pain, general undernourished appearance, mouth ulcers, anaemia or vitamin deficiency with fatigue, paleness, skin rash or bone pain, and in children, mildly bowed legs.

Although coeliac disease was first described in 1888, it was only in 1964 that researchers began to agree that it was caused by eating foods made from wheat.

Coeliac disease is known to be a genetically influenced condition which is caused by the gluten from wheat (see Chapter 6 for an explanation of gluten) chronically damaging the inside lining of the small intestine.

As recently as 1990 in Europe, and 1996 in the US, coeliac disease was considered quite rare and thought to begin in early childhood. However, in recent years, knowledge of the disease has dramatically changed with the discovery that huge numbers of people who do not show the traditional signs of coeliac disease are gluten-sensitive. A far wider range of medical conditions than was previously thought appear to be connected with gluten, and improve or even go into remission when gluten is removed from the diet.

It has also been discovered that it is not only the gluten from wheat that causes symptoms, but that from many other grains and some vegetables. In addition, dairy foods have been shown to cause symptoms. The inevitable conclusion is that all these are foods that have only relatively recently been eaten by human beings, and to which many of us have not yet become adapted in an evolutionary sense (see Chapter 5).

As researchers discover more and more conditions caused by these foods, they are beginning to recognise that coeliac disease is just one subset of a wide range of conditions and are calling for the name to be changed to 'gluten-sensitivity'.

Even within the coeliac disease subset, they are discovering how much more widespread this disease is than was previously thought.

Blood tests being used in the screening of six-year-olds in Italy are revealing antibodies to gluten in children whose symptoms have not yet begun to fully emerge.

Detailed information about the latest methods of testing for coeliac disease and the many other diseases now thought to be caused or worsened by gluten, such as certain forms of cancer, osteoporosis, brain disorders, intestinal disease and digestive disorders (for which the authors list an impressive number of scientific sources), is to be found in *Dangerous Grains* by James Braly and Ron Hoggan, published in 2002 (see References). The authors recommend a gluten-free diet in all cases and give case histories of people whose diseases have gone into remission by eliminating gluten.

However, they maintain that a gluten-free diet is considered very difficult, because people don't understand the range of foods which contain gluten and doctors don't understand that many people are extremely sensitive to even the smallest amount of gluten.

Examples are included of people suffering from coeliac disease in hospital being given meals which contain a small amount of gluten, because doctors think a completely gluten-free diet is unpleasant and feel they are depriving patients; a more liberal approach is considered more humane. There is also an example of one patient with coeliac disease, becoming sicker and sicker despite many years on a gluten-free diet, who discovered almost on the point of death that the medications she was taking contained gluten. No one had thought to point this out to her because it was not known that these tiny amounts of gluten could cause such problems.

The authors say that, to add to the difficulties of a gluten-free diet, the purification process which separates wheat starch from gluten protein is far from perfect. They recommend that people with coeliac disease and gluten-sensitivities should not eat wheat starch. If you have been on a gluten-free diet without success, or with variable success, starch could be the reason. The very simple method of testing for starch with iodine, as outlined in Chapter 8, would also reveal the presence of gluten. All people with gluten-sensitive diseases should be told of this method.

However, all the recipes in this book can be eaten with complete safety by people with coeliac disease or any other gluten-sensitive condition. Follow the delicious IBS Low-Starch Diet and you will never again need to worry about eating gluten.

4

Why has no other doctor told me this?

There is a huge diversity of opinion amongst doctors and specialists on the causes of back pain, and even more on the causes of IBS. As we have already discussed, most GPs do not recognise that the two conditions may be part of the same syndrome.

Doctors have difficulty with the diagnosis. It is therefore likely that each doctor or specialist will give you a different opinion. Your treatment will depend on who you see.

Typically, you will have suffered years of chronic backache and IBS before you get the correct diagnosis of AS – and this will usually only be made by the doctor when you begin to show advanced signs; that is, when disabling, degenerative spinal symptoms begin.

Even then, it is doubtful that any rheumatologist to whom you are referred will know how to alleviate the symptoms, other than by prescribing anti-inflammatory drugs, exercise and localised heat treatments. Even with drugs, they will not know how to prevent the relentless, degenerative spinal symptoms of AS.

Here is a quotation from a chapter contributed by the Director of NASS (the National Ankylosing Spondylitis Society) to a state-of-the-art book:

> Ankylosing spondylitis is such a variable condition that every patient's experience is different. The first major problem encountered by patients worldwide is misdiagnosis . . . The disease goes unsuspected, despite years of symptoms, either by the primary physician or by the specialists. Repeated visits to physicians lead to the suspicion of neurosis. The undiagnosed patient feels frustrated, isolated, and angry at being considered neurotic or a malingerer. After several years, some patients also experience additional loneliness due to the withdrawal of sympathy from friends and members of their family who begin to sympathise with the physician's misdiagnosis.

Upon diagnosis the patient is given only a brief description of the disorder, most of which is rapidly forgotten. The primary physician knows little about the condition and either cannot give advice or gives inappropriate advice. Even after diagnosis . . . the patient feels helpless and this feeling is reinforced by the family doctor informing him that, apart from anti-inflammatory medication, nothing can be done.

From 'Ankylosing Spondylitis – the patient's point of view', by Fergus J. Rogers, in *The Spondylarthritides*, edited by Andrei Calin and Joel D. Taurog, Oxford University Press, 1998. Reprinted by permission of Oxford University Press.

The misdiagnosis and mismanagement of IBS and AS

It is interesting that the myths and misconceptions about the two major early symptoms of AS, gut pain and backache, continue relentlessly. New research is funded for both conditions; new books are written every year, without revealing any new information or producing any solutions. As I write, a major research project at an NHS hospital into IBS is investigating 'The IBS personality'. Emphasis is always on emotional stress. 'Think of it as migraine in the gut,' one doctor said to me. 'It's as if you're crying inside . . .'

Specialists in back pain have many different theories about its cause and treatment. But on one subject they all agree: back pain is a twentieth-century disaster. The eminent orthopaedic surgeon Gordon Waddell, in his comprehensive book *The Back Pain Revolution* (Churchill Livingstone, 1998), says: '*Modern medicine has been very successful in treating many serious spinal diseases, but* [the] *traditional medical approach has failed with back pain . . . Chronic back pain and disability should be reducing, but instead the opposite is true. Why?*' He goes on to say that doctors do not really understand the cause of most back pain, and that most of the conventional treatments are ineffective. '*Indeed, many of the things we do may actually be worse than no treatment at all.*'

Physiotherapists have considerable success teaching specific exercises, on land or in the water, to stretch tight muscles, improve chest movement and strengthen muscles that help keep patients' spines straight and joints mobile. A regime of maintaining good posture begun in the early years of the disease, to prevent the forward-stooping posture of the spine, has been shown to improve life for AS sufferers. Some rheumatologists work with physiotherapists to help their patients in this way. But many people who have corresponded with me after being diagnosed with AS have been given no information about this by their rheumatologist, nor had any further help or advice other than to be told they will probably have to have hip-replacement operations and perhaps end up in a wheelchair. The only treatment on offer has been pain-relieving drugs.

It is a big mistake to think that drug therapy alone is appropriate for managing AS. Drugs are simply given to reduce the inflammation, pain and stiffness and to allow the patient to become more active.

Unless you were lucky enough in the past to be diagnosed correctly and then referred to Professor Ebringer's AS clinic, you would not have been given information by any other doctor about treating AS with a low-starch diet. Even this information is no longer available in the UK through the NHS, because Professor Ebringer's clinic has now been closed down, due to insufficient funding. Not many people realise that funding for such clinics often comes from private sources. Drug companies are always prepared to fund researchers who are using or researching their drugs. Professor Ebringer's dietary treatment is of no interest to them.

A few other reputable books written by doctors about arthritic diseases now mention the HLA-B27/*klebsiella* connection, and also recommend a low-starch diet, without any advice on how to manage such a diet.

But despite having published over seventy papers on his research, and conducted studies in ten countries over the last twelve years, Professor Ebringer's successful treatment of AS with the low-starch diet has not been accepted by the rheumatology world.

It is said that there was interest in the theory at one time, but research workers were not able to replicate the findings. I believe this is because they did not correctly understand the difference between carbohydrates and starch, and did not recognise the huge number of hidden starches in our food. They therefore found it impossible to correctly plan and implement a starch-free diet.

How do I know that this information is reliable?

If your blood test shows that you are HLA-B27 positive, you should discuss this with your doctor and ask his opinion. There is a list of some of the scientific papers written by Professor Ebringer and his colleagues, and other literature about AS, at the back of the book, to which your doctor can refer.

But you are also at liberty simply to try the IBS Low-Starch Diet yourself, as described in this book. You should be able to detect a difference in your symptoms within a relatively short period – say, two to three months, if not sooner. The IBS symptoms usually disappear within a couple of weeks.

The diet involves no dangerous drugs. You will suffer no dangerous side effects. You will feel remarkably healthy. The food is delicious and if you have a weight problem you'll find you're losing weight in a steady, healthy way.

Many AS patients report a huge change in their health and well-being within a short time. Once they try the diet, they are convinced. To their joy and amazement, relief from symptoms is often achieved in a matter of days, and they want to tell other sufferers about their results. It is no flash in the pan – the diet persuades the sufferer to stick with it, because of the relief.

Not only will you get relief from pain, but the IBS Low-Starch Diet will prevent the progress of the disease

A low-starch diet is the only method of treatment available at present which will give you remission of symptoms. Patients report that the inflammatory bowel symptoms disappear and their stiffness and joint pains fade away. You will not be cured – you still have AS. But if you are young enough, you will never experience the disabling degenerative spinal symptoms. And even if you have begun to show early signs of disability and stiffness, you will experience a remission of these (see the case histories, below).

Unlike the drugs which many of you take, and which cause terrible side effects, this diet will only make you feel healthier and more energetic. If you're overweight, you'll get slimmer and begin to look younger. But the most wonderful effect will be the remission of your symptoms.

Remember – there is no pressure for you to stick rigidly to the IBS Low-Starch Diet. You can stop at any time and go back to your normal way of eating. Many AS patients report that at first, the idea of giving up all the foods they love is unacceptable, so they go back to their previous diet. The resulting return of symptoms quickly puts them back on the low-starch diet. You may also feel so much better after a few months that you think you're cured and you can start eating normally again. All of us fall off the wagon from time to time. It's okay. When those AS or IBS symptoms return, don't feel a sense of failure. Just start again.

It may seem an appalling idea, to give up the starchy foods that are so delicious. But this book is full of recipes and substitute foods that are just as delicious. And remember – you don't *have* to do the diet. If you can put up with the pain, the bloating and the disablement, the side effects of the drugs and the prospect of a future in a wheelchair – *don't diet.*

I'm too much of a coward!

Some case histories and letters

Chris: who wouldn't take 'no diet will help' for an answer

Chris is an enterprising young man with a successful career in the film industry. In his mid-twenties he began to have trouble with one of his eyes, and iritis was diagnosed. At the time he was lucky enough to be seen by an ophthalmologist who told him that sometimes this condition was the precursor of an arthritic disease, ankylosing spondylitis, and that he should have a blood test to see if he had the HLA-B27 gene. When he proved to be positive, he was told that his chances of developing AS were nothing to worry about, as only 3 per cent of people with this gene go on to develop the disease.

But about a year later he began to get a very bad sciatic-like pain in his buttock and leg, with stiffness in his back, to the point where he could hardly lift himself out of bed. Thinking it may have been a strain from the gym, he went to the doctor, who referred him to a rheumatologist. X-rays and an MRI scan revealed that Chris's sacro-iliac joints showed signs of inflammation and some minor bone changes which, along with his genetic make-up and the iritis, led to a classic diagnosis of AS.

'*Of course I was horrified, as this is generally thought of as a chronic, progressive disease that can end up putting people into wheelchairs. I was told it can be extremely painful and that I would gradually lose the flexibility of my spine and develop a curved spine and stoop. Once, I remember seeing a man who had obviously been afflicted with AS for many years, bent over double, walking with a stick whilst looking into a mirror to see which way he was going!*'

The only advice Chris received was that he would have to take extremely powerful anti-inflammatories for the rest of his life, and exercise to try to maintain as much movement as possible. '*They told me that there was no cure and that no one knew exactly why this condition starts up in otherwise perfectly healthy young people. You can imagine how I felt – in my twenties with my career just beginning to take off – to be told this!*'

Chris was not prepared to be so easily beaten. He was also not convinced that medication was the only solution. He began scouring the Internet and gradually began to find bits of information about *'certain research papers that had been done by a Professor Alan Ebringer in London'*. He contacted me by phone in May, 2001, after hearing that my IBS Starch-Free Diet would work for AS, and from then on, as he says, *'I did a strictly no-starch diet for five months (just eating meat, fish, vegetables, salads and fruit) and in no time at all, the pain dissipated and eventually vanished, only to return again if I had a heavily starchy meal. I used to live on pasta, which explains perhaps why my first attack was so bad.'*

Chris has discovered that he is now able to eat bread in normal quantities, but he still finds that pasta, potatoes and rice start to bring back the beginnings of the old pains again. He says he recently experimented and ate three bowls of pasta over three consecutive days, and, *'Lo and behold, the pain started to return. This was my sign to cut it out there and then, and direct proof that the diet and the theory is correct.'*

In August 2001, he went back to the rheumatologist who had diagnosed him, and who had also told him that NO diet would help. The rheumatologist checked Chris for flexibility and was absolutely astonished that he could find no deterioration whatsoever. Chris then told him that he had been on the diet, and, in Chris's words: *'His whole attitude completely changed. He was charming and delighted: I had never seen a consultant so excited before! He said that on the basis of what he had just seen, he would start recommending the diet to his other AS patients.'*

Chris asked him whether it could be sheer coincidence that his symptoms had mostly disappeared. The rheumatologist said he thought it most unlikely. In his opinion, AS pain can be pretty severe when you first get it, and it rarely, if ever, goes into complete remission so soon after onset. The only explanation for the lessening of pain and stiffness was *'that the diet had put the AS into remission'*. Chris says, *'He even dictated these very words into a tape recording machine for his own records!'*

In October 2002, Chris wrote to tell me that *'AS no longer features in my life whatsoever. I have been painfree . . . since I last was in touch with you, I have been able to eat bread in normal quantities. I stay off the pasta, spuds and rice . . . which I hardly miss now . . . I am also never tired any more after meals as I used to be after eating those heavy starches.'*

Chris doesn't take any pain-relievers now, not even paracetamol. He believes he is *'100% cured – back to normal!'* Despite Chris's wonderful remission of symptoms, none of us will ever be 100 per cent cured. However, he is so enthusiastic about the diet and Professor Ebringer's findings that he says, *'The man deserves the Nobel Prize! Ask yourself this: in the past, haven't many of the greatest ideas from Galileo to Einstein been the ones most beautifully simple and seemingly obvious? Penicillin, perhaps the most important drug of our era, was, after all, discovered by accident!'*

When I last heard, Chris was still in complete remission.

Two letters typical of many I receive from people who suffered for years:

Dear Carol,

It's with gratitude that I've chosen to write this brief message of thanks. The revelation that is your book has given me confidence in my physical ability to meet the demands of business and life in general.

I was diagnosed as a sufferer of Reiter's syndrome at the age of eighteen in 1969. Throughout the period since, I have endured chronic back pain and bouts of severe arthritic flare-ups affecting major joints and surrounding soft tissue. The most recent episode occurred in January of this year [2005] after a slow build-up over the Christmas period. I had a return of all the typical symptoms so I immediately implemented my regular regime of eliminating almost every food other than fish, salad, fruit and vegetables from my diet, which provided some tentative relief.

Through pure coincidence my wife was attending a naturopathic physician at the time and just happened to ask the doctor if she knew anything of Reiter's syndrome and whether any more recent developments had occurred in its treatment. The doctor detailed some of her knowledge of the still relatively little-known complaint and then simply quoted the name of your book. We purchased the book that day and when I took it home to read was amazed and excited to find not only a specific reference to Reiter's but the coincidences between my symptoms and those you had written about.

To cut a long story short, I went to my doctor and took the blood test. He was at first a little cynical so imagine his surprise when he learned, and had to inform me, that I tested positive to the HLA-B27 gene. Even before testing I had already begun following your diet with positive results. You can imagine, however, my feelings of elation when I learned of the diagnosis and, for the first time in nearly forty years, having the knowledge to explain the cause and effect of my illness.

From about two to three days after I began following the dietary advice in your book the pain began to diminish. I have been almost entirely pain-free and without medication for over a month and I am also confident that I will remain so. If I have any temporary twinge I can always identify it with a calculated risk I have taken the previous day to experiment with foods outside your guidelines.

What is also quite amazing is that apart from total relief from my arthritic problems, I hadn't realised the extent to which I was tolerating pain and discomfort in my digestive system until it was also gone. This was just an absolute unanticipated bonus. At fifty-four years of age I am again the same weight and size as I was in my mid-twenties. This is also a bonus.

I have purchased your book for three other people including my son and my sister (who has since been diagnosed with the gene and suffers back and other related pain). I cannot recommend your book too highly to anyone who feels it may help. It has opened the door to new possibilities for me.

Regards,
Robin
(Australia)

Dear Carol,
Thank you so much for emailing me back. I had been sick for ten years on and off with iritis in my left eye, sore neck, aches and pains, nausea and fever and general unwellness. I had been to numerous doctors and specialists, but no one could find anything wrong with me.

I was at my wits' end when my sister saw your article in the NZ Herald June 15 2004. Then I bought your book and I knew straightaway I had AS.

It was confirmed through a blood test, which came up positive although, like you, I had no signs of arthritis or spinal degeneration. I decided to go on the AS diet and cut out all starch from my diet. I have been on the diet for six months and have never felt so well. All signs of iritis, aches and pains etc. have now disappeared. I can finally get on with my life (I have a husband, two sons – twelve and nine – to look after). It's just so wonderful to be well.

Thank you Carol for writing your book and making people like me aware of this illness. Who would have thought by altering your diet you could be well again?

My brother has also been diagnosed with AS. I am sure my late mother had it as well.

You suffered dreadfully for many years and it must be wonderful for yourself to be well too. I am quite strict on my diet but do miss potatoes. I may introduce a little bit of starch food in the next coming months and see how I get on.

The recipes in your book are just great.
Kindest regards,
Marie
(New Zealand)

Danny: struggling from denial to dealing with the disease

Danny contacted me from Texas just as he was about to graduate from college. A couple of years previously he had begun noticing stiffness in his neck and (as he called it) his tailbone. His doctor arranged for him to have the HLA-B27 blood test, which was positive, and then referred him to a rheumatologist.

In Danny's own words, '*The rheumatologist told me I probably had AS and that all I could do was stay in shape, and that the worst case scenario was that I would have to get my hips replaced in the future!! Needless to say, I never went back to him again! I didn't believe I could have some weird disease. So I had two MRIs (magnetic resonance imaging) done; they showed nothing really. A neurologist referred me to a chiropractor. The chiropractor actually helped me. He told me I needed to get in shape and he did adjustments to my spine and neck, and the pain almost completely went away . . . I was also eating a lot better.*'

However, Danny's neck stiffness never completely went away. But he thought to himself, '*See, Danny, you didn't have any kind of disease . . . Anyway, a year goes by and I start eating whatever I want, and start getting lazy . . . Well, in September, right before the World Trade Center attacks, I started getting stiffness again in my spine and neck. That is when I started to get really sad, thinking, "Oh my gosh, maybe they were right, and I have this AS thing." Then I met Chris on the net, and he gave me a lot of hope and referred me to you and Dr Ebringer's findings . . . I started cutting starch out and did notice a difference, although it seems like it comes and goes. Some weeks will be good and other days will be stiff, and it is frustrating . . . I am willing to cut starch completely out. I have only been on this diet now for like a month, and don't get me wrong, I have noticed a change, but should it be completely gone by now?*'

I was able to reassure Danny that he should give it more than a month's trial, and his symptoms improved. But a year later he contacted me in a panic. He had developed pain and redness in one eye and had heard that this was part of the AS syndrome and could result in blindness. I told him to go straight to an ophthalmologist and say he was HLA-B27 positive, which he did. Luckily, he didn't have iritis (sometimes also called uveitis), which is the eye condition that can cause blindness, but a less serious condition called episcleritis. But episcleritis takes a long time to disappear, and I had many despairing e-mails from him as he struggled to come to terms with the many symptoms of AS. '*They say AS affects about one in one thousand people, and sometimes I can't help but think that one person had to be me out of those one thousand . . . I know that there are people out there that are far worse off than me, and I have no right to complain, yet I still sometimes think I have it bad, when really my AS pains are fairly minimal.*'

Danny is finding the diet hard going. He says it is such a drastic change from the way he used to eat, but notices how quickly the symptoms return when he eats starch again. Like most young people, he doesn't know what goes into the food he eats. He has begun testing with iodine, but is dismayed at the number of foods in which he finds starch. He says the diet has helped him tremendously, and he hopes everyone who has AS takes the same measures, but he knows this will be a lifelong struggle.

'This is my life . . . I am twenty-three now and am still a bit bitter about the whole thing . . . but it has really tested my soul and I have to pull through and be grateful about all the other things in my life that are good. My view on AS is, I can beat this . . . I am not going to be a pity case, and I am not going to let this disease get the best of me. There is a way to control it. My pain is mainly in my neck and middle back. My head [used to feel] *like it weighs a thousand pounds on the pillow. With the low-starch diet I rarely feel this weight any more.'*

Some people with AS don't suffer as much as Danny; some suffer more badly. But everyone would agree with his final word: *'Let's tell these scientists to hurry up and create something to counter this autoimmune disease . . .'*

Because the diagnosis of IBS is such a vague term, there may be a number of causes of the condition, and the low-starch diet may not work for everyone. However, many women suffering from IBS have written to me over the years to say how much the low-starch diet has helped them. Here are extracts from a poignant letter from one of them.

Colette: now living a life she thought she never would have

Dear Mrs Sinclair,

I am very ashamed to say it is over two years now since you were good enough to write and tell me when your book The Sinclair Diet System *was due to come out.*

It is completely inadequate but all I can really say is 'Thank you'. . .

I am now living the life I thought I would never have. I can go out to eat with my family, something I could never do before as I had too much pain and discomfort.

Reading about you when you were young was almost like reading about myself. I always felt the trouble and pain I had was due to what I ate. I just did not know how to start. All through my life from being very young my doctor just said it was all nerves and in my head, once suggesting I needed to see a psychiatrist as I had a persecution problem.

From that time on I decided to save my breath. Until years later when I had married, moved and had a different doctor! Then I got an appointment with a gastroenterologist at the R—O— Hospital who did not tell me I was mad but that it was irritable bowel syndrome. That was in 1987.

I do not have the words to tell you how bad my life could be at times in the past and how good it feels now. My mother says I am a different person, relaxed and calm. It is so easy when you are not in pain almost all the time.

As I said before it is completely inadequate. All I can say is 'Thank you' to you . . . for giving me a life I thought I would never have.

Yours sincerely,
Colette

Since I discovered the real cause of my IBS, I have tried to contact everyone who wrote to me to let them know they should ask their GP for a blood test to see if they have the HLA-B27 gene. Colette phoned me recently to say she has had the blood test and is not HLA-B27 positive, but that the diet still works for her.

George McCaffery: from despair to success story

George first contacted me in 1999, to tell me that the low-starch diet worked for AS. Without George I would probably never have heard the name ankylosing spondylitis, or discovered that I also had the disease. George has been on the diet almost as long as I have. He calls it the 'secret' diet because, in his own words, 'doctors keep it a secret'. His story is remarkable and an inspiration to us all.

'Around about the age of twenty-six I began to experience what I believed to be groin strains and thigh strains. My GP gave me pain killers/anti-inflammatory drugs and told me to rest. I eventually persuaded my GP to refer me to a specialist as these apparent injuries persisted and worsened. At age twenty-eight I was seen by an orthopaedic specialist in Newcastle who diagnosed a spinal instability needing a bone graft from my pelvis on to my spine.

'I was admitted to the Freeman Hospital in Newcastle around 1978. I was prepared for theatre, i.e. shaved from toenails to ears – and starved. The morning of the operation the surgeon came to see me and asked how I was. He couldn't believe it when I told him I was feeling great. He lifted one leg at a time and dropped them – no problem. The stiffness had disappeared. He asked me to get out of bed and touch my toes – no problem! He then decided not to operate. Boy, am I pleased he called it off! Strange! I crawled into that bed and jumped out!'

What George didn't know was that the pre-operative starvation had deprived his gut of starch and had quickly caused the sudden loss of pain and stiffness. But after this George went through a number of years sometimes feeling okay, sometimes feeling terrible. In 1982 he went to live in Singapore and began experiencing worsening pain and stiffness. His doctor in Singapore prescribed anti-inflammatory tablets which George describes as *'great big pink things, as big as a door-stop'*. As well as the drugs, George was trying anything and everything. *'During this period I tried physiotherapy, a sports physician in Guildford who injected a solution radially through the muscles on either side of my spine (this is more painful than having AS but doesn't last as long), a blind mystic healer in Indonesia, acupuncture, massage . . .'* You name it, George tried it.

'Around 1986 my GP in Singapore had some more X-rays taken and blood tests. He then told me I probably had something called ankylosing spondylitis, a progressive bone disease which had no cure, but which could burn itself out. I should continue to take the anti-inflammatories. But I was having major problems with my stomach. At times I couldn't tell if the pain was from my stomach or back (sounds crazy doesn't it?).'

Still in search of a cure, George visited Guy's Hospital in London. *'Someone had told me that a hospital in London was the place for AS, and Guy's was the only one I had heard of. I met a really good rheumatologist there, who told me the recommended treatment for AS was NSAIDs [non-steroidal anti-inflammatory drugs] and, for longer-term results, sulpha-salazine. He also mentioned that there was a school of thought that said diet may come into it. Of course I thought nothing of this. I had a bone disease, and what could diet have to do with it?*

'Around 1988 someone told me they had read that a doctor at the Middlesex Hospital was doing research into AS. I phoned the Middlesex from Singapore. I was desperate at this time, in a lot of pain and contemplating having to give up work. I was told by a nurse in Rheumatology, "Oh, that will be Doctor Ebringer." Eventually I was able to speak to Dr Ebringer and told him of my situation, and asked if there were any research programmes I could be a part of. I persuaded him to see me and came across in February of 1988.

'Doctor Ebringer examined me (I crawled on to the table). He looked at my X-rays and sent me for blood tests. In March of 1988 I went back and he told me, "You have AS. You are HLA-B27 positive and your ESR* is ninety-eight." I said, "That's just great, Doc. I've already been told the first bit. I don't know what the other numbers mean. Just don't tell me you can't do anything for me and to keep on taking the tablets!"

'He said, "Not exactly, but I will tell you – you can help yourself." He then explained the low-starch diet/klebsiella theory and gave me the Middlesex sheet of what to eat and what not to eat.

'I have to say, at this point I was thinking, Oh no – a bloody quack! However, I said, "Okay, you tell me my problem is starch. Not another bit of

---

* ESR (erythrocyte sedimentation rate): a blood test which gives an index of inflammation. Elevated levels indicate disease activity.

starch will pass my lips!" (Probably a threat to expose his stupid theory.) I went on a bacon and egg diet as it was the only thing I could think of that didn't have starch in it.

'Three days later, I woke up (I can remember exactly where I was, the Grand Hotel in Brighton) feeling great! I phoned Ebringer, elated, and told him what was happening. He said, "Good. Stick with it."

'GOOD! I couldn't believe it was that simple! Why had no one told me before?

'The rest is history. Once I found the problem, I could control it – look carefully at the contents of things I ate. The psoriasis I had on my elbow and in my ears cleared up in a week or so. I kept on visiting Dr Ebringer's clinic in London whenever I passed through the country, and at the last count my ESR was eighteen.

'I now have a lot of friends with AS through a website at www.kickas.org, which is a NSD [no-starch diet] site, with a lot of people with similar experiences to mine from going on a low-starch diet.'

George is being slightly modest here, because the rest of his history is that as a result of the low-starch diet he began to feel so well that he went on to become the managing director of a public company on the stock exchange in the UK. Then he started his own company in the USA, built it up, opened offices in other countries, and finally sold it recently for, as he says, '*a few million quid. Which I definitely could not have done without the secret diet*'.

5

But don't we *need* to eat a high-carbohydrate diet?

Well – that's what we've been told most of our lives. But in fact there is actually no specific dietary requirement for carbohydrates in the human diet. I was amazed when I first came across this information in textbooks on nutrition. Various nutritionists phrase it differently, but the information is always the same: the exact carbohydrate needs in the body have not been established; there is no recommended daily allowance for carbohydrates; the actual amount of carbohydrates required by humans for health is zero.

When nutritionists talk about the 'requirement' of certain foods in the body, they mean the specific level required to maintain health. No specific level of carbohydrate has been arrived at because the body can (and does in certain populations) function healthily without carbohydrates, or with minimal amounts. So no level of carbohydrates has been identified as being essential to health.

To understand these staggering statements, we need to understand the different functions of carbohydrates and proteins in the body. Carbohydrates provide energy for the body, in the form of calories. Proteins do the job of renewing, maintaining, regulating and making the body work. Without protein, no life can exist (the word 'protein' is derived from Greek and means 'holding the first place'). But if enough energy is not provided in the form of calories, the proteins can't get on with their essential work.

However, carbohydrates are not the only food group that provides energy. The fat in animal proteins actually produces 2.25 times as much energy per pound as do carbohydrates. So we don't actually need carbohydrates, as long as we include some fat or oil in our diet. You may have heard of the 'ketogenic' diet. This is where the principal energy source is fat, rather than carbohydrates. It's what the Eskimos lived on successfully for years. It is even more astounding to consider the diet of a Central African tribe called the Masai. They exist on milk, meat and blood, supplemented by concoctions made from the bark of trees and certain roots. This may seem a repulsive diet to us; however, they maintain good health, and unlike us Westerners show no signs of deficiency diseases.

But carbohydrates are a good source of energy and we love them. The ideal amount of carbohydrate in an average diet – perfect for keeping the body in great condition – is from 50 to 100gms daily, depending on the individual. But this doesn't have to be in the form of starch. The low-starch diet will give you sufficient carbohydrates in low-starch vegetables, fruit, desserts, cakes, ice-cream, wine and beer. (Yes – alcohol is not only permitted but recommended, in moderation, on this diet!)

Nevertheless, a diet much higher in carbohydrates – especially the really starchy ones – is the standard advice given by nutritionists and doctors. The belief that it would be better for health if meat intake was reduced and seen as an added extra to the meal, rather than its central feature, has been the standard dietary advice from British health authorities since the late 1940s. I have come across some quite bizarre reasons for recommending a reduction in protein. It has long been known that a high-protein diet helps withstand cold temperatures, but I even read in one book on nutrition that a diet high in protein was no longer needed because we all now live in heated houses!

Not only do health authorities recommend a high-carbohydrate diet for normal diets and weight-loss diets, but also for people with IBS, constipation, arthritis, obesity, gastrointestinal problems, heart disease, high blood pressure and diabetes – all the chronic diseases of modern man.

But any doctor today will tell you that our diet is causing an epidemic of these diseases – and they don't know what to do about it.

You mean a high-carbohydrate diet is wrong?

Doctors and nutritionists beg us to eat the low-fat, high-carbohydrate diet. Patients try even harder to follow the rules, eating a diet rich in potatoes, low-fat pasta, rice, bread, toasted breakfast cereals with added vitamins and minerals. We increase our intake of low-fat foods like yoghurts and desserts with added modified starch to replace the fat (the very description 'low-fat' almost guarantees that the food will contain additional starch).

And what happens? We get fatter and sicker.

The patient gets the blame, of course. Doctors believe we are not sticking to the diet. But it is the low-fat, high-carbohydrate diet that is the cause.

Health officials have consistently targeted the wrong food group. Instead of fat, they should be identifying the high-carbohydrate diet as the cause of obesity.

It is interesting to see how seriously people have taken the advice to eat less fat. For example, in 1910, the average consumption of butter per person in the US was 8.3 kilogrammes. By 1990 it had dropped to 2.0 kilogrammes. In 1988, in an effort to reduce obesity and the many associated health problems, the American public were officially advised to eat less fat and more carbohydrates. Food manufacturers obliged with vast numbers of low-fat products. Surveys showed that the American public cut back dramatically on the amount of fat in their diets. But instead of obesity rates reducing, research now reveals that there was a 32 per cent increase in the following ten years.

You don't have to be a doctor to see that obesity is on the increase in this country – just look around during your weekly trip to the supermarket. You'll also notice that most of the obese shoppers also have other health problems: they often limp, or walk with sticks. Many of them have disabled badges on their cars. Obesity is always the sign of other health problems – one of the most incapacitating of which is arthritis. A recent report by a committee of MPs said: *'Obesity in England has reached "shocking" levels contributing to 30,000 deaths a year ... Unless more is done to combat the problem, one in five men and about a quarter of women could be obese in three years' time.'*

Increasingly, doctors in America, Canada, New Zealand and Australia are questioning the failure of the low-fat, high-carbohydrate diet.

Some are putting their patients on exactly the opposite – a low-carbohydrate diet – with spectacular results. You may have heard of these diets. They're sometimes called 'celebrity diets' because so many people in showbiz recommend them for losing weight and feeling great. People also wrongly refer to them as 'high-protein' diets – which they are not. They are simply *adequate*-protein diets, in which the correct balance for the human body has been restored. And they really work!

It's quite simple, really: the modern high-carbohydrate diet provides too much energy in the form of starch. Our bodies don't need it and can't process it. It gets stored as fat in our bodies and lies undigested in the gut, providing a food source for bacteria, causing disease, fermentation and pain.

In a normal digestive system, most people do not completely digest starch, even if only a small amount is consumed. In order to process a high-carbohydrate diet, the body must produce excessive amounts of insulin. This, in turn, produces insulin resistance, followed by the requirement for ever more insulin to keep the system going. Elevated insulin levels are now being recognised by a small number of doctors and researchers as the underlying cause of obesity, heart disease, high blood pressure and diabetes – in other words, the common diseases of the Western world.

I believe the problems of our modern diet would be solved if only nutritionists properly understood the difference between carbohydrates and starch. As you will see in Chapter 6, all plant foods are carbohydrate – but not all carbohydrates are starch. Too much starch in the diet is what is causing such an epidemic of obesity and disease in our world. This book is not about weight loss, but if you're overweight, you'll certainly lose weight and feel fantastic on the IBS Low-Starch Diet.

Why isn't the high-carbohydrate diet working?

The high-starch carbohydrates – the grains and cultivated root foods which are now such a large part of our diet – are quite new in evolutionary terms. For over seven hundred thousand years our ancestors ate a diet of primarily meat, fat, nuts, wild roots, fruit and berries. They did have other uses for carbohydrates – they fermented them, fuelled their fires with them, built with them and fed them to their animals.

Recent discoveries of prehistoric human fossils have astounded scientists. These were the hunter-gatherers – people who lived mainly on meat, roots and berries. Instead of small, stunted people with signs of disease, their skeletal remains reveal that these hunter-gatherers were tall and lean, with well-developed, strong, dense bones with no signs of osteoporosis, and sound teeth.

They did not suffer from arthritis and had little evidence of chronic disease. Whole family groups have been discovered, consisting of grandparents, parents and children, showing that life expectancy was longer than at any other period prior to our own.

Not only did they live longer, but they were taller – considerably taller – than the humans who followed them: the agriculturists.

Around ten thousand years ago humans learned to grow their own food, enabling them to give up their nomadic lifestyles and become farmers. Life became more sophisticated. Food storage and cooking improved.

Grains, which could be stored the whole year round and eaten in so many ways, were cultivated and cross-bred to produce the wheat, barley and oats we know today. Even then, grain foods were the convenience foods of their day. Bread could be carried around, eaten cold in the field or added to other foods.

Lentils, which had been unpalatable or toxic when raw, were dried and became an important cooked addition to the diet, often replacing meat.

Roots, previously eaten only in small amounts and then usually raw, were cultivated to become larger and starchier. All these foods could be stored throughout the winter and eaten when meat was in short supply.

Without doubt, these developments were responsible for a cultural leap forward: instead of spending most of their time hunting for food, people had time for leisure pursuits – art, music, learning, all the things that led to civilisation.

But human health declined. The skeletal remains of these people are considerably shorter than the meat-eaters, with much less-developed skeletons. They show signs of malnutrition, stunted growth, brittle bones, osteoporosis, arthritis, tooth decay and many chronic diseases.

The early Egyptians had the perfect diet. Why, then, did they have modern diseases?

Egypt was one of the earliest agrarian societies. The average diet was just what is recommended today – rich in fruit and vegetables, some fish and poultry but very little red meat. They also consumed olive oil, goat's milk and wine. But the most important part of their diet was bread made from unrefined, stone-ground wheat and barley. Sounds ideal. They should have been extremely healthy. But the Egyptian mummies and the surviving papyrus writings reveal just the opposite. All the chronic diseases that doctors worry so much about today, and which are such a financial burden to our Western nations (in 1994, back pain alone cost the UK £6 billion in medical bills and loss of earnings, rising by £0.5 billion every year), also plagued the Egyptians.

Egyptian mummies have preserved a fascinating record of the disastrous change in health that occurred when our ancestors began eating a high-carbohydrate diet. In the skeletal and tissue remains we have an enormous repository of medical information. And in the accounts of the daily lives that survive on papyrus and stone, we have documentary evidence of the diet they ate, and of illnesses that were common.

The change from a diet high in protein to one high in carbohydrates caused a decline in health all over the world. Despite modern nutritional advice, we were never meant to eat a diet composed of 60 to 75 per cent carbohydrate. In the US, the recommendation from some nutritionists is as high as 85 per cent. Our digestive system, with its single stomach, has evolved to eat a diet of predominantly meat, supplemented with roots, shoots, berries, seeds and nuts. To properly digest a high-carbohydrate diet we would need a number of stomachs – like a cow.

The change to a carbohydrate diet happened too suddenly for our digestive system to adapt to it. The excessive insulin and insulin resistance that a high-carbohydrate diet causes is seriously damaging to our health. However, the diseases that this causes are chronic rather than terminal. In other words, we don't immediately die of our high-carbohydrate diet – we simply live in agony, having survived to pass on our genes to our children.

If the diseases caused by the high-carbohydrate diet killed us when we were young, we would not have lived long enough to have children, and the diseases would probably have died out too. But the advance of medical science has meant that we live on into old age, getting crippled with arthritis, getting sicker and sicker with diabetes, heart disease, obesity and brittle bones.

Where our Western diet goes, people get sick

These chronic diseases are now emerging in populations whose primitive lifestyle has suddenly changed to that of the modern Western world.

The Inuit people (Eskimos), American Indians, Aborigines, Pacific Islanders, Maoris – peoples from isolated populations who have begun eating a Western diet only within the last century – are all now stricken with these diseases. The Pima Indians from central Arizona lived on rabbits, lizards, cactus fruit, beans and squash for centuries. Within twenty-five years of adopting a Western diet, 50 per cent of the over-thirties and many teenagers suffer from adult-onset diabetes and obesity. They are also particularly prone to AS. In some Native American populations, nearly 50 per cent of the whole population gets diabetes.

The Inuit are now amongst the sickest people in Canada, with high rates of all modern chronic diseases. Right up until the early twentieth century, the Inuit thrived in the coldest, most arduous climate in the world. Arthritis, heart disease, strokes, cancer and high blood pressure were almost unknown among them. The Inuit diet was the subject of a fascinating study by Canadian Vilhjalmur Stefansson. In the early 1900s he travelled for years throughout Canada studying their health, noting that they lived on a diet high in animal fat and virtually devoid of carbohydrates. They had no access to grains, vegetables or fruit, except a few berries, and lived almost entirely on fish, seal and whale blubber. Their consumption of calories was around 2,500 a day, of which 75 per cent was fat.

In 1929, Stefansson and another scientist checked into the Bellevue Hospital in New York City to carry out an experiment. They lived for months on a diet of nothing but fresh meat and fat, during which time they were monitored by doctors. At the end of the experiment both men had lost six pounds (2.75 kilos) in weight, felt extraordinarily well, looked younger and had amazing vitality. The experiment made headlines all over America – the evidence was incontrovertible. But like a number of other similar experiments and papers written by scientists on the importance of a low-carbohydrate diet, the medical profession ignored them, or dismissed them as cranks.

Not everyone is unlucky enough to get sick from eating a high-carbohydrate diet. Perhaps, somewhere in the past, their ancestors' digestive systems adapted to it. Many people appear to have no health problems living on a vegetarian diet, especially when they're young. The high-carbohydrate diet that most children exist on – pizza, chips, cola drinks, biscuits, cakes, cereal and toast – seems fine, until they're in their late twenties. Then, for many, their diet and their genes begin to catch up with them. In general terms, by the time they're in their forties, about one-third of the population in the Western world has some of the chronic diseases now known to be associated with a high intake of starch.

How did the myth of the healthy high-carbohydrate diet begin? And why?

It started because of a religious belief. In the early 1800s a former Presbyterian preacher, the Reverend Sylvester Graham, toured America, giving lectures on the virtues of giving up fats and meat, and eating coarse, wholegrain breads. The famous Graham cracker is named after him.

To a certain extent his ideas were based on the dietary problems that had begun to emerge as a result of the Industrial Revolution. The milling and refining of flour had made bread relatively cheap and easy to produce, enormously increasing the intake of starch in the average diet, while at the same time reducing the quality of the carbohydrates eaten. Graham's mistake was to urge people to adopt an unbalanced diet by discouraging the eating of meat and fats.

However, his ideas were seized upon by Sister Ellen White, later known as Mother White, one of the early leaders of the Seventh-Day Adventist Church, who are opposed, on religious grounds, to eating meat. In 1866, this zealous lady founded the Western Health Reform Institute at Battle Creek, Michigan.

The people who flocked to Battle Creek were already experiencing gastrointestinal problems. The discomfort they felt from the normal amount of carbohydrates they'd been eating was soon greatly increased by the high-carbohydrate 'health' diet. But Sylvester Graham and Mother White insisted the problems had been caused by eating meat, and that when they had flushed their systems of 'protein poison' they would become healthy. Desperate for a cure, the poor patients stuck to the high-carbohydrate diet, with disastrous results.

Mother White's ideas continued to be preached with evangelical zeal throughout America. Half a century later, huge numbers of people had been persuaded to eat these 'health foods'. Increasing numbers of patients were arriving at the Western Health Reform Institute to be cured of dyspepsia, indigestion, constipation and other gastro-intestinal problems.

Along came Dr John Harvey Kellogg, also a Seventh-Day Adventist. Dr Kellogg would not eat meat under any circumstances. He had been hired by Mother White to manage the institute and his presence was mesmerising. His fanatical preaching drew crowds to hear him thunder from the pulpit: 'Steak is sin!' Among other benefits, he claimed that a vegetarian diet reduced sex drive. Sex, even between married couples, should be rationed, he maintained, so as not to weaken the system. His meetings were more like old-time temperance meetings than nutrition lectures. People fainted, cried, broke down in hysterics and signed up to obey Dr Kellogg's rules of diet and self-denial of meat, alcohol, tobacco and sex.

By now, so many susceptible people were suffering from the effects of the meatless, high-carbohydrate diet that Dr Kellogg turned the Western Health Reform Institute into the Battle Creek Sanitarium. Thousands of patients swarmed to this Sanitarium and paid large sums to undergo a regime of strict vegetarian meals, exercise, laxatives and five-times-a-day enemas. Daily menus consisted of dishes guaranteed to cause the greatest possible gastrointestinal discomfort to people who already had problems digesting starch: Bean Tapioca Soup, Nut Lisbon Steak, Corn Pulp, Bran Biscuits, Gluten Mash. The longer the patients stayed, the worse they would feel and the more extreme would become the treatments.

But the Sanitarium patients were the rich and famous of their day. News spread far and wide about Dr Kellogg's treatments. It became fashionable to take the cure at the 'San'. Kellogg began to become very wealthy, especially when he invented a granola-like, ready-to-eat breakfast cereal, not only for his patients but for Adventists everywhere, who shunned the traditional American breakfast of ham and eggs. When his brother Will began the mass manufacture of another of John's inventions, the dried, toasted breakfast cereal which they called 'corn flakes', their fame and wealth was assured.

By the mid-1930s, America was in the grip of health-food mania. Other cereal companies began to spring up, some founded by former patients of Dr Kellogg, such as C.W. Post, who marketed a cereal substitute for coffee, and the famous Grape-Nuts breakfast cereal. Health-food shops promoting the vegetarian way of life were opening everywhere. Digestive problems had now become a national mania. Chronic diseases such as arthritis, obesity and diabetes were on the increase.

It is fascinating to note that in 1977, an American researcher, Professor Finegold, and his co-workers carried out research on the rates of faecal microbial culture to be found in subjects on a high-carbohydrate/low-protein diet, as compared with those on a low-carbohydrate/high-protein diet. The high-carbohydrate people were all Seventh-Day Adventists – ideal subjects because of their vegetarian diet. The findings showed that for the people on the low-carbohydrate/high-protein diet, the average number of *klebsiella* bacteria was 700 per gram of faeces. However, for the Seventh-Day Adventists, the average number of *klebsiella* bacteria was 30,000 per gram of faeces. How many of these people suffered from IBS/AS symptoms was not measured, but the rate of these symptoms in vegetarians is very high.

In the 1960s and 70s, the health-food industry was given an enormous boost by ideological young people, especially hippies, rebelling against the ecological problems caused by industrial farming and the mass manufacture of foods. Like so many worthy ideals, it has now become a mass-market industry, polluted by the profit motive. The health-promoting qualities of these foods are dubious at best, and the adherents are seldom healthy.

The real junk foods of your diet

Today, new cereal products are developed by the major cereal manufacturers every year. No longer eaten just for breakfast, ready-to-eat breakfast cereals have become a basic diet for many people because of their convenience. Many are sugar- and chocolate-coated, and we binge on them because of their sweet taste. Made into 'high-energy, low-fat' bars and cookies, they are heavily marketed as 'ideal for school lunch boxes'. Added to yoghurts and ice-creams, they contain more 'empty' calories. Recent studies on the increase in the content of sugar in breakfast cereals found that some contained more than 50 per cent table sugar.

Ready-to-eat breakfast cereals are the most unnatural and highly processed of the foods we eat. The manufacturing process produces cereals that are higher in starch than the original grains, but lower in most other nutrients. The raw cereals are parboiled, cracked, extruded, flaked, popped, puffed, shaped, sugar-coated or shredded. The oil is removed by a combination of heating, pressing and solvent extraction. At this stage there is very little nutritional value left, so manufacturers spray them with vitamins and minerals to 'enrich' and 'fortify' them, and then make extraordinary claims for their health-giving properties.

However, the nutrients added are vastly inferior to the nutrients lost in the processing. During the so-called 'enrichment' process, only four of the more than two dozen essential nutrients that are lost in the processing are restored. Furthermore, substantial amounts of added fats and sugars are included. Nevertheless, advertising, news media, magazines, books and self-styled nutrition experts have elevated breakfast cereals to an unprecedented position in our diet. Consumers believe they are nutritious. In fact, they are the real junk food of our diet.

Before the craze for ready-to-eat toasted cereal changed the breakfast habits of the Western world, an adequate-protein meal, usually including eggs, was the breakfast of choice. It is a sobering fact that despite the claims which nutritionists now make for the health-giving properties of a high-carbohydrate diet, the diet of the Western world was dramatically changed solely because of religious fanaticism. As someone said, 'They meant to do good, and they did well!' Now the cereal industry is one of the largest and most profitable in the world.

And the number of people suffering from chronic diseases caused by the excessive consumption of cereals increases massively every year.

The importance of protein

Protein is essential for life. Without it, we would die. Protein is made up of amino acids, which are often called the 'building blocks' of life. There are nine amino acids that are essential for human development and thirteen that are non-essential for humans, but some of these are essential for animals.

If one essential amino acid is missing from your diet, a certain protein or proteins will not be formed. In an adult this means you will enter a state of 'negative nitrogen balance', while a child or infant will cease to grow. Each specific protein performs a specific function in the body. One protein cannot and will not substitute for another.

Proteins continuously form new tissues in the body, from infancy to adulthood. They also maintain body tissues, replacing blood cells, the cells that line the intestine, protein lost from the body in perspiration, hair, fingernails, skin, urine and faeces. Proteins regulate all body functions, such as blood clotting, water balance, oxygen balance. Many of the hormones that regulate body processes are proteins. Antibodies which protect the body from infectious diseases are proteins.

But not all proteins are created equal

Some proteins of certain foods are low in or completely devoid of some essential amino acids. This is why protein quality is so important in human nutrition. Plant foods often contain insufficient quality of four essential amino acids. Cereals are lacking in one essential amino acid and beans (pulses or legumes) are lacking in another. If the right plant foods are eaten together or within a few hours of each other, a better protein balance can be achieved. For example, Mexicans eat beans and corn, Indians eat wheat and legumes. But a better combination is plant food and animal protein together, such as bread and cheese, or cereals with milk.

Another problem with plant protein is its lack of digestibility. Although most animal proteins are about 90 to 95 per cent digestible and therefore can be properly absorbed to do their work in the body, the digestibility of some plant proteins may be as low as 73 per cent.

Protein malnutrition is the world's most disastrous dietary problem. There is a whole range of health problems caused in underdeveloped areas of the world because not enough high-quality protein is available. The worst of these is a condition called kwashiorkor, which in the Ashanti dialect means 'disease of a child when another is born'. Children fed low-protein, starchy foods such as bananas, yams and cassava after weaning develop this condition, which causes drastic physical and mental problems and will usually lead to death. We've all seen photos of little children with the huge, bloated belly which is a sign of kwashiorkor. This can be reversed when adequate protein is added to the diet.

Elderly people who do not eat a diet adequate in protein will experience exhaustion, mental confusion and the delayed healing of wounds.

In general, the proteins of animal origin – eggs, dairy products, fish, poultry and meats – provide mixtures of amino acids that are best suited for human requirements. These foods are excellent sources of high-quality protein. Eggs in particular contain all the essential amino acids in sufficient quantities and balance to meet the body's requirements, without excess.

If we all ate a diet adequate in high-quality protein and low in starch, it would transform our lives.

6

More about starch

The most common question I am asked when I say I can't eat starch is, 'What is starch?' Even some doctors and dietitians seem to be vague about exactly what starch is and the difference between carbohydrates and starch.

Most people are confused about the difference between carbohydrates, starch and gluten. And this is a pity, because many people suffering the symptoms of IBS and AS who have tried eliminating wheat and/or gluten, and still have symptoms, come to the conclusion that diet is not the answer. If you are unknowingly eating starch, you naturally conclude your symptoms are being caused by something else.

Even dietitians make mistakes. I have seen low-starch diets prepared by hospital dietitians which include lentils in the list of permitted foods, because they are high in vegetable protein. But they are even higher in starch!

Even when dietitians understand the differences in an academic sense, they don't warn against the huge number of hidden starches that are now being added to the foods in our supermarkets. You might think you're eating a protein meal when you eat chicken casserole, for example. But if carrots and peas are included in the recipe, the casserole contains starch. Even without vegetables which you know to be starchy, if a food additive such as acetylated distarch glycerol is added, the meal includes starch. Protein foods such as low-fat yoghurt usually contain starch. In fact, the words 'low-fat' almost always mean that starch has been added.

It is also surprising that there are many people who know so little about food that they don't know the difference between carbohydrates and protein! Most of these are probably young people who have never had to cook or buy food – but many young men develop AS and are overwhelmed by the difficulty of having to learn what to eat when they go on a low-starch diet.

You may be saying, 'But how will I ever be able to tell the difference? I've never had a lesson in food chemistry in my life!' It's actually very easy. You don't need to memorise lists of starchy foods. There is a simple test that even a child can do, which immediately tells you if food contains starch. We'll come to that in Chapter 8.

People with coeliac disease who can't eat gluten could learn to be absolutely sure they weren't eating wheat flour if they were taught how to test suspect food for starch. If you wish, you don't need to read this chapter any further to be able to identify starch. Just turn immediately to Chapter 8. But if you are interested, read on.

What's the difference between carbohydrate and starch?

All starches are carbohydrates, but not all carbohydrates are starch. For example, honey is a carbohydrate, but it is not starch. Grapes are carbohydrate but they are not starch. Bread is both carbohydrate and starch. Lentils are both carbohydrate and starch.

Experts tend to forget this vital difference. Most foods which they refer to as carbohydrate are, in fact, basically starch. That's why you'll often hear them referred to as 'refined carbohydrates'. The starch has been separated, through various processes, from the carbohydrate.

Carbohydrate is the term used to describe all parts of the plant. But in fact plants are made up of cellulose, sugars and/or starch. The cellulose part is the framework of the plant which contains the sugars and/or starch. We can't digest the cellulose. It passes right through our digestive system. It's excellent fibre, which of course we also need to regulate our digestion.

When the plant is processed or refined, the cellulose part is often discarded and the result is that we eat far more starch than nature intended, because it is easier to eat the food without the cellulose content. Grains of wheat are ground into flour. If it is white flour, the bran of the wheat, which is the cellulose part, is discarded. Sugar cane, which is perfectly healthy in its natural state, is turned into grains of sugar. It's far easier to eat sugar in its refined, processed state than to munch through the sugar cane. But this is the problem.

If you had to eat as much sugar cane as you get in the form of sugar in the average plate of cereal or packet of biscuits, you wouldn't be able to do it. In its raw state, the sugar cane would be too filling. If you had to eat as much unrefined wheat grain as you get in the form of flour in the average cake, you couldn't possibly manage it. Everything that happens to a plant after it is harvested is a form of processing – or refinement. If we ate it in its natural state, it would be unprocessed, or unrefined.

It is the starch, or the refined carbohydrate, that causes what experts now call 'carbohydrate craving'. I prefer to call it starch addiction, because it is the starch rather than the carbohydrate that causes the craving. All our processed foods that slip down so easily and that we can binge on so frequently are 'refined carbohydrate' – in other words, starch.

Starch

All food is divided into two basic groups: proteins and carbohydrates. Animal products are basically protein; plant products are basically carbohydrate. Some plants also contain proteins, and animal foods also contain glycogen, which is sometimes called animal starch because it is composed of glucose (don't worry about it at the moment) and is a form of carbohydrate in fat.

Plants store carbohydrates in the form of sugars, or saccharides, in different combinations of simplicity or complexity.

The very simplest are called monosaccharides, which means 'one sugar', and are the building blocks from which the more complex carbohydrates are built. The monosaccharides are glucose and fructose (found in fruit) and galactose (found in milk).

The next most complex are called disaccharides, or 'two sugars': these are sucrose (found in sugar cane and sugar beet), which is a combination of glucose and fructose; lactose (found in milk), which is a combination of galactose and glucose; and maltose (found in germinating cereals), which is a combination of two glucose sugars.

The most complex of all are the polysaccharides, or 'many sugars', which are a combination of all the above and others not mentioned. These are called starch and are found in a wide range of grains and vegetables, and a few fruits.

I have discovered that the more complex the saccharide is, the longer it is cooked or processed and the more I eat – the more trouble it causes me. I get more pain, bloating and joint pains from eating polysaccharides, for example, than from eating disaccharides. Monosaccharides don't cause me any problems.

It's taken me years to understand which saccharide is which, and which ones cause my symptoms. To help me remember, I think of them like this:

Mild-mannered monosaccharides

These are the sweet-tempered, gentle sugars that won't cause you any pain.

- Glucose – found only in grapes.
- Fructose – found in fruit.

- Galactose – found in milk. (Galactose is not available individually, but only in conjunction with lactose.)

Dodgy disaccharides

You have to be careful of these sugars – they're devious and can be dangerous if you eat too many, especially when they're cooked for a long time.

- Sucrose – found in all forms of ordinary sugar, brown and white.
- Lactose – found in milk.
- Maltose – found in germinating cereal seeds and cooked vegetables.

Painful polysaccharides

These will cause you real trouble. They're the ones that are most likely to cause the pain and bloating of IBS and the symptoms of AS. Although they're saccharides, they don't look or taste like sugar. Collectively they're known as:

- Starch – found in all grains, lentils and most vegetables, but not in most fruits.

What's the difference between carbohydrate and protein?

I've already covered this in Chapter 5, but just in case you didn't read it, here it is again: carbohydrates and proteins have different, but interdependent, tasks to keep you going. Think of your body like a car. Carbohydrates are the fuel – they provide energy for the body, in the form of calories. Proteins are like the mechanic – they maintain, regulate and renew the engine, electrics, chassis *and* bodywork. Without sufficient protein, you'd be a malfunctioning, battered wreck and no matter how much energy you put into it, your body wouldn't work properly.

But carbohydrates are not the only form of energy: fat in animal proteins actually produces 2.25 times as much energy per pound as do plant carbohydrates. So as long as you include some oil or fat in your diet, you actually don't need plant carbohydrates.

However, carbohydrates are a good source of energy and we love them. The ideal daily amount is from 50 to 100gms. But this doesn't have to be in the form of starch. The IBS Low-Starch Diet will give you sufficient carbohydrates in ice-cream, salads, low-starch vegetables, fruit, low-starch desserts, cakes, wine and beer.

What's the difference between starch and gluten?

Gluten is not starch – it is a plant protein found mainly in wheat. Rye also contains gluten, as do oats and barley. Corn and rice are low in gluten. When liquid and other ingredients are added to wheat flour and the dough is kneaded, the gluten develops and gives bread elasticity and strength.

Coeliac disease is a well-known condition in which the lining of the gut is damaged by gluten, preventing the absorption of essential nutrients. People who have coeliac disease, sprue (similar to coeliac disease) or gluten allergy cannot eat food containing gluten. There is an increasing variety of gluten-free foods on the market.

It is interesting to note that recently some doctors have discovered that the endomysial antibody test (EMSA) for coeliac disease has revealed that a high number of patients with obscure symptoms who have never previously been diagnosed with coeliac disease have, nevertheless, tested positive. All have improved on a gluten-free diet.

How does our body know the difference between protein and carbohydrate?

The difference is incredibly important, and our body knows it. Within hours, the food we eat, whether from plants or animals, turns into flesh and blood. We take this for granted, of course, not thinking about the processes going on in our body. But such a complex transformation can't be achieved unless the food has undergone a drastic breaking-down process. And during that transformation, our body takes note of the different foods we eat, and processes them in different ways. We call this transformation digestion.

Digestion involves both physical processes (such as chewing and peristalsis (gut movement) and chemical processes (such as digestive enzymes) to break down the food particles into smaller particles and convert them into even smaller molecules and atoms, known as nutrients.

Different digestive enzymes break down different foods

Digestion begins even before we put food in our mouths. Just the smell of delicious food is enough to 'start the juices flowing'. We have fewer digestive juices for plant foods than for animal protein, but of these digestive juices, the first – and the one we are probably most aware of – is saliva, or salivary amylase, which digests carbohydrate. That's why we need to chew our food thoroughly to get it as well digested as possible before we swallow it and send it on its way. The other digestive juice for starch is pancreatic amylase, which doesn't develop until we are around six months old. This is why babies can have gastrointestinal problems if they are given starchy foods too early.

Ultimately, all digestible carbohydrates are broken down by the pancreatic hormone insulin into the monosaccharide glucose, which has been described as the 'chief source of fuel for the metabolic fire of life'.

Proteins, which do the job of renewing and maintaining the body, are more complicated and are converted into a number of different amino acids. Each specific protein performs a specific function in the body. Basically, proteins and fats perform five different functions, including producing energy, and are broken down by a number of different enzymes.

Ultimately, everything is broken down into the smallest possible nutrients, which pass into the bloodstream and are then absorbed into the cells of the body. This is known as absorption. People who suffer from malabsorption problems, such as the inability to absorb vitamin B12, which is sometimes diagnosed as pernicious anaemia, develop deficiency symptoms and must be treated by injections directly into the bloodstream. Their ability to absorb through normal digestion has, in some way, been destroyed.

Certain foodstuffs which cannot be absorbed, such as fibre, pass through the digestive system and perform the job of keeping it clean and on the move.

After being mixed with saliva in the mouth, our food begins its long and complicated journey through a series of tube-like organs, which are basically the stomach, and the small and large intestines (or gut). All the way along it is being subjected to the most amazing array of digestive enzymes (including hydrochloric acid in the stomach, strong enough to dissolve iron nails and other metals!) and processes which mix and break down the food. If we could see this taking place in a laboratory, we'd be amazed at science in action.

Digestion is very interesting – or very distressing, depending on whether yours is 'good' or 'bad'. But however effective your digestion is, you will not entirely digest all the starch you eat. There is always partially digested starch in the gut, no matter how small an amount you have eaten. And this is where most of the bacteria live, on the partially digested starch.

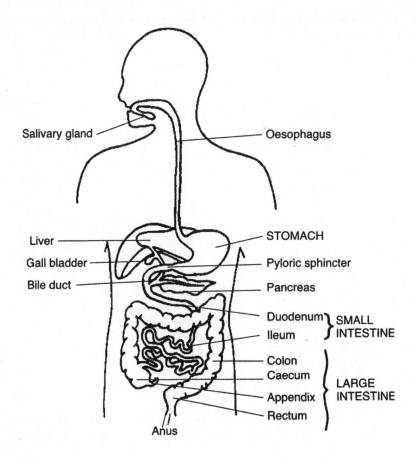

Salivary gland

Oesophagus

Liver

STOMACH

Gall bladder

Pyloric sphincter

Bile duct

Pancreas

Duodenum ⎫ SMALL
Ileum   ⎰ INTESTINE

Colon
Caecum

LARGE
INTESTINE

Appendix

Rectum

Anus

The digestive system

Most bacteria are helpful – they're the benefactors of mankind; without them no life on earth could exist. But some bacteria are the agents of death and disease. During digestion, much bad bacteria is destroyed by digestive enzymes such as the hydrochloric acid in our stomach. But then our body's immune system takes over, deciding which of the bacteria that survives is good, and which should be destroyed.

When a bad bacterium, such as *Klebsiella pneumoniae*, which resembles the HLA-B27 gene, takes up residence in the gut of people who have this gene, then in order to destroy it, the immune system mistakenly begins to destroy its own body cells. This is the cause of our symptoms of IBS and AS.

Discover the level of starch consumption you feel comfortable with

In my search for a cure, I'd been told I had an 'IBS personality' and that this was the cause of my symptoms. I'm sure my medical notes from that period are littered with descriptions of me as an anxious, neurotic patient. But the amazing disappearance of my symptoms after giving up not only wheat flour but all grain foods convinced me that my problems were caused by food. Although after a year or so of giving up grain foods my symptoms returned, nevertheless, that was the longest time I could ever remember being free of symptoms in my adult life. So I wasn't about to give up on diet.

If you're eating starch in food regularly, the symptoms of pain and bloating are almost always present. It is therefore impossible to determine whether it is the starch or other foods causing it. But after I had eliminated all grain foods in my diet, I knew what it was like to be free of pain and bloating, and I was determined to feel like that again.

Not to know why certain foods cause your symptoms is confusing and dangerous. It's not safe to rely on a list of which foods to avoid, because it is not the individual food that causes our problems, but something *in* the food. And that something has to be based on a scientific principle.

In the early days of my diet, before I had discovered this, there were many times when I felt terribly discouraged at the return of symptoms. It obviously wasn't only food made from grains – after all, beans and lentils were amongst the worst culprits. I began to realise that it wasn't enough to know that certain foods caused my symptoms. I had to know why some apparently random foods did so when others didn't. What did these foods have in common? I decided it could only be starch. I knew potatoes, rice and corn (maize) also contain starch, so I gave them up too – and the symptoms went away again.

For quite a while all went well. Then the symptoms came back. But I couldn't believe it was my starch theory that was at fault, so I didn't give up. After a lot of thought and testing, I realised that every time I ate cooked vegetables, the symptoms returned. Raw vegetables and cooked or raw fruits caused no problems. But why?

Then I remembered a very crotchety chemistry teacher – about a thousand years ago, it seemed – teaching us that vegetables contain starch and drawing diagrams on the board showing how the cell walls of vegetables are changed during cooking, releasing the starch. If the vegetables are eaten raw, the starch travels in little waterproof envelopes through the digestive system and is not released. Fruits, on the other hand, contain starch when they are green, but upon ripening the starch turns to fruit sugar (fructose). This is why, if they were properly ripened, I could eat both raw and cooked fruit.

There are exceptions to this rule – some fruits that contain starch and some vegetables that don't – and I will list them in the next chapter. And I still had more to discover about starch. But at this stage my diet consisted of meat, cheese, eggs, salads, fruit, ice cream, yoghurt, cream, milk and starch-free sweets such as chocolate, as well as coffee, tea and alcohol – and I felt great.

And then my symptoms returned. I was devastated. I searched every item of my diet for possible hidden sources of starch, and it occurred to me that perhaps some tablets I had been prescribed might contain starch to bind them. I asked my doctor and the local chemist. Neither could give me an answer. In those days, only the active ingredients in pills and tablets had to be listed in the information about drugs. So I phoned the drug companies. It took a lot of fast talking to convince them I was not a reporter trying to dig up dirt on them, but in the end they confirmed my suspicions. Most pills and tablets contain rice or maize flour. Even these tiny amounts of starch were causing the return of my symptoms. Luckily my doctor could prescribe liquid versions of the medications I needed, so the symptoms disappeared again.

In recent years I've been getting letters from readers suffering from IBS and AS, and have begun to realise that perhaps I am particularly sensitive to starch. Some people tell me they can eat certain starchy foods, but not others. I will list all the foods I am unable to eat, but I now believe it is up to you to discover the level of starch consumption you feel comfortable with.

People experience IBS and AS symptoms in different degrees

It has always been known that people suffer from IBS and AS in variable degrees. This is dependent on the number of copies of the HLA-B27 gene you have in your body. I'm sure this is also the reason why some people are more sensitive than others to starch.

However, there is also the inescapable fact that sensitivity can increase, due to the way our immune system works. As already described earlier in the book, when the immune system first detects an 'invader' in our body in the form of a bacterium or virus, it sends out the 'troops' (antibodies) to destroy it. If the invader resembles one of our genes, the immune system accidentally begins to destroy its own body cells. The appearance of the invader is carefully stored in the immune system's memory, so that next time the invasion occurs, the immune system can be ready to attack just that little bit faster. Each time there is another invasion, the immune system becomes quicker off the mark.

There is nothing we can do about this – at the moment. Science may, in the future, discover a way to retrain our immune system to recognise only the invader and leave our body cells alone.

But from the earliest onset of your symptoms, your body has been attacking itself. This would have happened whether you had eliminated the invader (the *klebsiella* bacterium) or not. But many people tell me how quickly they experience the return of symptoms if they go off the diet.

Before I understood that my symptoms were the result of an autoimmune disease, I used to think that every time I experienced the return of symptoms more severely, it was because, having discovered what it was like to be free of pain, I had become increasingly sensitive to the return of symptoms. In a way I was right. If you've never lived without the symptoms at some level, you don't know what it's like to be without them. When at last you become free of pain, you certainly notice when it returns!

7

Which foods contain starch?

Grain foods (cereals)

Contain starch both when cooked and when raw. They are the starchiest and also the most common and widely eaten foods all over the world. Cereals are a major part of a normal diet: breakfast cereals, bread, cakes, pastries, batters, vegeburgers, pasta – all contain grain starch, usually in the form of wheat flour. Most people eat cereal, in some way or other, at every meal. Some people seem to eat nothing but!

Rice is one of the most important cereal grains in the world and provides most of the food for over half the human population. However, it is the only major cereal that is largely consumed as harvested (after hulling and usually polishing), whereas wheat and other grains are usually highly processed before eating – a factor which reduces their nutrition and adds to their indigestibility. Other grain foods high in starch are corn (maize), barley, oats and rye.

I cannot eat *any* food containing starch from grains. Even a very small amount causes IBS pain and bloating within a couple of hours. The joint pains of AS begin the next day.

Vegetables

Most root vegetables, such as potatoes, parsnips and sweet potatoes, are very high in starch. Turnips and swedes may not contain enough starch to cause problems for many people. Many green vegetables release starch when they're cooked but not when they're raw. A few vegetables do not contain starch, even when they're cooked. Cooked spinach, asparagus, fennel and mild onions seem to be reliably starch-free. Broccoli is very low in starch. Cooked mushrooms and tomatoes I eat with caution – not too often or too much.

It's not easy to tell which contain starch and which don't just by looking at them, but see Chapter 8 for a simple way of testing to see which foods contain starch.

Fruit

Contains starch before it is ripe. When ripe, the starch turns to fruit sugar, or fructose. Fruit containing only fructose can be eaten both cooked and raw – with the exception of bananas, which are very starchy and cannot be eaten either cooked or raw. Rhubarb, which is really a vegetable, also contains starch.

Citrus fruits contain starch in the white pith. This is released when the fruit is squeezed or crushed, or when the skin is eaten. Obviously, less starch will be released if the fruit is very carefully peeled. It will depend on your tolerance levels whether you are able to eat and drink citrus fruits and juices, but if you find symptoms returning, I would advise elimination.

Avocado, which is really a fruit, can be eaten if on testing it does not contain starch. But I have learned in recent years that fruit that is picked before it is ripe and stored in cold-storage until it is put on the supermarket shelves will contain starch. Most fruit contains starch before it is ripe (melons may be the exception – I have never found any melon to contain starch). When fruit is properly ripened – especially on the tree or vine – all the starch turns to fructose.

Sugar

Sucrose (ordinary table or cooking sugar) does not contain starch but it is a dodgy disaccharide. Therefore I can eat it in small amounts. For example, I can eat one meringue (made the traditional way without cornflour, of course) but not two. If I eat too much sugar, I will experience some bloating and a little pain. The longer sugar is cooked and the more it browns, or becomes caramelised, the less easy it is to digest, because digestive-resistant starches are produced during the cooking. However, as with all sugars, this depends on how much you eat, and how often. Many of you will be able to eat sugar without adverse effects. Maple syrup is sucrose but I enjoy it on bacon and eat it almost every day for breakfast as a way of including carbohydrate with a protein meal.

While we're talking about sugars, here's an interesting piece of information about honey. Health foodies have maintained for years that honey is far better for you than sugar (sucrose). But most chemists shake their heads in disbelief, because the nectar which the bees collect to make the honey is made up of small amounts of glucose and fructose, but is largely sucrose. And no one ever recommends sugar as a health food! However, while the nectar is being processed through the bee's honey sac and deposited in the hive, it is being pre-digested and broken down into fructose and glucose. The hard-working bee has done us the favour of turning a disaccharide into mild-mannered monosaccharides, making it much easier to digest than ordinary sugar.

Milk

Dairy foods do not contain starch, but they contain lactose, which is a dodgy disaccharide. When milk is correctly digested, the lactose is broken down into glucose and galactose. But if you can't digest it properly, then it ferments in the gut causing symptoms of IBS – a condition known as lactose intolerance. Other metabolic disorders that are known to be caused by milk in some people are milk allergy, milk intolerance, galactose disease and milk anaemia.

Lactose intolerance is most likely to occur in African, Eastern European, Middle and Far Eastern people or their descendants, who for reasons not fully understood do not secrete lactase, the enzyme needed to digest milk, after their mid-teens. However, in the process of making cheese and yoghurt, the lactose has already been broken down into a digestible form by bacterial action, which means that often people with lactose intolerance can eat these foods. This is why yoghurt is frequently found in Indian recipes.

Lactose intolerance can occur following gastric surgery, and as one gets older. But it is known that it can also develop with diseases such as ulcerative colitis, enteritis, Crohn's disease (all of which are also called inflammatory bowel disease), gluten enteropathy and cystic fibrosis.

I ate dairy foods for years before finally I had to cut down, probably due to getting older (the digestive system gets less efficient as we get older). Now I have problems with cow's milk products but find that I can eat small amounts of cheese (such as Roquefort, feta, Parmesan, chèvre and halloumi) and yoghurts made from goat or sheep's milk, or mozzarella made from buffalo's milk. These milks contain less fat, but despite having combed all sorts of books on nutrition, I cannot find out whether they contain less lactose. Therefore I don't know why I can tolerate small amounts of them, and not cow's milk. But as they are recommended for people with lactose intolerance, I suspect they are lower in lactose.

I can also eat low-fat ice-cream (as long as it doesn't contain modified starch). But, unfortunately, most low-fat yoghurts contain modified starch.

Modern storage systems increase starch content

Supermarkets need to delay the ripening of fruit, in order to prolong shelf-life. Most of the fruit we buy these days is picked before it is ripe and has been kept in cold storage for some time in order to delay the ripening process. The irradiation process used to prevent or slow down ripening is another factor. For example, I find that most supermarket-bought apples I test these days – even the sweet, red varieties – show the presence of starch. This wasn't so in the early years when I began my diet.

Whatever the technique used, much fruit sold in supermarkets shows signs of starch when tested, which means that the fruit has not been able to ripen naturally, allowing the starch to turn to fructose. This is especially true of imported fruit, or fruit eaten out of season.

The exceptions to this appear to be soft fruits, melons and grapes. Raspberries, strawberries, blackberries, black- and redcurrants and cherries have never caused me any trouble. Even when these fruits are frozen they are fine. I presume it is because they are picked when they are ripe and can't be cold-stored over a long period. Melons seem to contain no starch, whether they are slightly green or really ripe. Grapes are also free of starch, except for the skins of red grapes, which contain some. I eat red grapes only in moderation. The other exception seems to be dried fruit. Presumably this is because the ripening doesn't need to be delayed. There is a wide variety of delicious dried fruit available these days which I often eat, in preference to fresh.

When I first began my diet I ate all fruit (except bananas) without any qualms. However, a couple of years ago I had an unpleasant experience when eating nectarines. For most of the summer I had tested and eaten this delicious fruit without any problems. But towards the end of the summer I bought some which, although they looked very rosy and ripe, were too hard to eat. I put them on the windowsill to allow them to ripen further, and discovered within a couple of days that they were rapidly developing bruised spots and had become suddenly very soft. Without bothering to test them I ate a couple, and within hours had very bad IBS pain and bloating. At that stage, cursing myself for not having done so earlier, I tested them for starch. I was horrified to find they contained as much as bread! I knew I was in for a miserable night, but it was far worse than I could have imagined. I became so ill with the pain that at about three a.m., my husband phoned for an ambulance and I was rushed to hospital. My bowel had gone into a loop, causing a blockage – a volvulus – which can be very dangerous (the same sort of thing that happens to a hose, causing a blockage). Luckily I had taken Epsom salts earlier in the evening, and this began to flush through my gut and relax the loop. When the doctor examined me he could still feel the volvulus, but by that time I assured him I knew I would be all right, and he let me go home.

Most of you may not be badly affected by fruit that is slightly starchy. But for those of you who have to be extremely careful, my advice is always to test before eating.

Starch is now added to almost every processed food

You can't live on starch. Starch by itself adds no nutritional value to your diet, except in the form of calories. It's the carbohydrate content of starchy food which contains vitamins and minerals. However, one of the most identifiable characteristics of starch is that it is an excellent glue. (I really don't want to bad-mouth starch – it's not its fault I can't eat it – but whenever I'm tempted to feel sorry for myself, I just conjure up an image of a large bucket of pale, gluggy wallpaper paste. Ugh!) It is therefore enormously useful to food manufacturers because it is the most efficient way to thicken food and provide the basic structure of much of the food eaten throughout the world.

Starch is invariably added to low-fat food because when fat is removed from foods such as ice-cream and yoghurt, the food will not thicken properly. Manufacturers add modified starch to give the required consistency. It is included in protein foods such as sausages, hamburgers and processed meats to stick them together – and it is used in foods such as grated cheese or sliced, pre-cooked meats as a coating, to *stop* them sticking together. It is often added to pre-prepared meals such as curries, simply to improve the appearance of the food, by preventing sauces separating in the pack. It is also included in manufactured foods which do not normally need to be thickened, such as chutneys or yoghurts, to cut down the natural thickening time in the processing. It is used in most medicines to bind them into tablets and pills. Starch saves money for the producer.

There are many types of starch used in processed food which go under different names. In most countries they are usually identified simply as 'starch', 'modified starch' or 'modified food starch'. Natural starch can be as commonplace as wheat flour, cornflour, arrowroot, maize flour, potato flour or rice flour. But modified starches have been changed by chemicals, or other processes, to perform better as a thickener than natural starch. Sometimes they are not even identified as modified starch. Maltodextrin is one example. This is a partly converted starch which when tested with iodine goes very black indeed. These starches are only used by commercial producers.

Babies have trouble digesting starch

Before the age of four months, infants have only a limited capacity to digest starch. A baby's ability to digest starch increases slowly, and even up to six months of age is only partially developed – the reason why the recent addition of so much modified starch to processed baby food is a bad idea. When babies eat food containing starch which they cannot properly digest, they may suffer various gastrointestinal problems, including colic. Babies can get colic for other reasons too – even when they are being breastfed only. But mothers should be aware that the increasing use of starch in the diet of babies when they are too young is commercially driven, and can cause problems.

We are now eating starches once not considered fit for human consumption

Some years ago an EU directive extended the range of permitted starches added to foods. In addition, the EU does not require starch to be identified in the ingredients list.

Most responsible manufacturers still include modified starch in the list of ingredients if it is included in their food. You will often see cornflour, maize or potato starch, or modified maize or modified potato starch, listed.

However, starches that were once not considered fit for human consumption in Britain are now added in highly modified forms to processed foods. These are permitted in foods for infants and young children, classified as weaning foods, and for special medical purposes.

I have discovered starch in yoghurts described as 'low-fat natural yoghurt containing nothing but milk and bacteria'. This could be especially dangerous to people suffering from coeliac disease.

Here is a list of starches that do not have E numbers and can legally be added to foods without being identified. Although these starches are generally recognised as safe for people with normal digestion, it is not known whether a significant increase in consumption would constitute a dietary hazard. Therefore, there are limitations on amounts that can be added to food. But if most of the food you are eating contains amounts of these, the build-up could be hazardous, even if you can normally tolerate starch.

Acid-treated starch
Alkaline-treated starch
Bleached starch

Oxidised starches
Monostarch phosphate
Distarch glycerol
Distarch phosphate A esterified with sodium trimetaphosphate
Distarch phosphate B esterified with phosphorusoxychloride
Acetylated distarch phosphate
Acetylated distarch adipate
Acetylated distarch glycerol
Hydroxypropyl starch
Hydroxypropyl distarch glycerol
Hydroxypropyl distarch phosphate
Phosphated distarch phosphate

Reproduced from *E for Additives* by Maurice Hanssen (Thorsons, 1987).

New evidence that starch can be harmful in human nutrition

There is much new evidence emerging to show that the new processing of starches and the additional use of starch is certainly harmful to many people. Until the 1980s, it was believed that starch was an easily digested food which was totally absorbed by the human digestive system. However, in the late 1980s nutritionists and scientists were beginning to have doubts. In June 1989, the University of Saskatchewan in Canada hosted a symposium to discuss starch in human nutrition. Many new papers on starch were presented. In her introduction to the symposium, Alison M. Stephen of the Division of Nutrition and Dietetics, College of Pharmacy, University of Saskatchewan, said:

> *During the 1970s, considerable research had been devoted to dietary fibre and its role in prevention and treatment of disease. But by 1980, it was becoming clear that some of the effects attributed to fibre might in part be due to starch, which is present in many of the same foods. The decade of the 1980s, therefore, saw an increased interest in the importance of dietary starch for human health and an exploration of the mechanisms by which starch might act at various levels of the gastrointestinal tract and elsewhere in the body. The fate of starch in the gastrointestinal tract emerged as a new area of study for the nutritionist and physiologist, as well as for the microbiologist investigating its fermentation in the large intestine ... Malabsorption*

of starch in the small intestine was discussed, including the emergence of the term 'resistant starch', that component which passes into the large intestine because of its resistance to hydrolysis and absorption in the small intestine. This was followed by papers on the fate of starch in the large intestine, the characteristics of its fermentation, and its effect on colonic function.

Starch and its behaviour in the human gut is now a major subject of scientific concern. However, most research on starch digestion has been conducted on people with normal digestion. The papers presented at the Saskatchewan symposium were no exception. The relationship of starch to diseases such as IBS and AS was not understood at that time, or discussed. More research is emerging about the problems of starch – especially grain starch – and the diseases of the Western world which may be directly attributed to it. We have not heard the last of this subject.

These thickening agents are safe

I have noticed since I wrote my first book that the addition of modified starch in certain prepared foods, especially ice-creams and chilled or frozen desserts, has declined. Manufacturers are increasingly using gelling agents such as xanthan gum (E415), guar gum (E412), locust bean gum (E410), carrageenan (E407), agar (E406) and pectin (E440a), none of which contains starch when tested with iodine.

Although you might think that these additives sound unnatural, they are in fact modified plant carbohydrate and are classed as 'fibre'. Carrageenan, for example, is a naturally occurring food gum obtained from seaweed, which is rich in minerals and vitamins. Pectin is a naturally occurring gelling agent found in fruit. I have no trouble eating foods with these thickening agents.

Coffeemate, which I use now that I don't eat dairy foods, is a good example of why we need to know what all those E numbers mean. I have friends who are shocked to see me putting something so 'unnatural' into my coffee. But here is what those E numbers on the Coffeemate jar mean, in the order they come on the label:

Glucose syrup (a monosaccharide)
Hydrogenated vegetable fat (vegetable oil)
Acidity regulators E331 (a form of citric acid which occurs
    naturally in citrus fruits, used to prevent discoloration of

food), and E340 and E452(i) (prepared from phosphorus, a nutrient required for every cell and fluid of the body and essential to combine with calcium for strong bones and teeth)

Calcium carbonate (we are all encouraged to consume more calcium)

Milk proteins (no lactose here)

Emulsifiers E471 and E472 (prepared from glycerol, a normal product of digestion, and acetic acid, which is from vinegar)

Colour: E101 (riboflavin or vitamin B)

So Coffeemate is a perfectly wholesome, lactose-free alternative to milk. This is an example of how E numbers can fool you.

8

How to identify starch in your food

The most common high-starch foods have a starchy look – they're usually pale and thick! Keep that in mind and you'll find it easy to recognise the foods most likely to cause IBS and AS symptoms. But it's not so easy to recognise starch in other foods.

Often when I thought I had eliminated every possible source of starch from my diet, the dreaded symptoms would return and I would be desperate again. There seemed to be no answer to identifying starch in some foods, except to eat them and suffer. And then my friendly local chemist reminded me of the easy test for starch: simply drop iodine on to a sample of the suspect food. (Don't eat the sample!) If it contains starch, the colour of the iodine will change. For most starchy foods, the iodine will darken from orange to shades ranging from inky-blue to black. Needless to say, I tested all sorts of food immediately. Flour, bread, cakes, potatoes and rice go a very dark blue-black colour – almost like carbon. The dark blue-black colour is a sign that these starchy foods are the amylose starches.

On other starchy foods, the iodine may go a very dark reddish-brown colour. These are the amylopectin starches, often found in the skins of fruit and the insoluble component of carbohydrates. They may not cause symptoms of IBS and AS in many people. However, they both cause the return of symptoms for me. (Interesting aside: amylodyspepsia is the medical name for the inability to digest starchy foods.)

You don't need to remember these names, but if you are as sensitive as I am to starch, you will want to watch out for any change in the colour of the iodine drop, from dark bluish-black to dark reddish-brown.

Raw sliced vegetables show signs of starch by going greyish around the edges, where the cell wall has been damaged by cutting. This is not enough to cause problems for most people.

On meat, cheese, eggs and animal products, the iodine colour remains unchanged (it may tend to go a little darker as it dries). The same should be true of most fruits if they are naturally ripened, except bananas, which in varying degrees, depending on how ripe they are, turn really dark when tested, proving they're full of starch.

Unfortunately, I sometimes still discover new sources of starch in foods. This is where the iodine starch test is a great help. If the starch content in the food is significant enough to cause IBS and AS symptoms, it will show up. If any food you test disagrees with my findings – i.e. if you discover it contains starch even when I have said it doesn't – then go by your starch test.

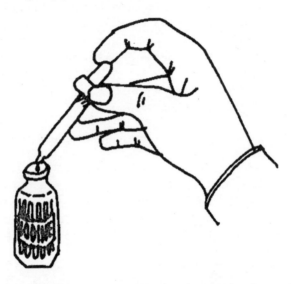

Test food separately. Do not eat tested food or iodine.

Buy a small bottle of iodine from the chemist and an eye-dropper. In order to see how really starchy food reacts, try the test first on a small piece of bread. Drop a small amount of the iodine on to it and watch the drop turn almost black. That is your benchmark. Nothing will go blacker than food made from grain flour. Every time you want to find out if food is safe to eat, drop the iodine on to a tiny piece of the suspect food, then wait a few minutes to see if the iodine changes from its normal orange colour. If you wish, you can dilute the iodine by up to 30 per cent with water before using it. This makes no difference to the colour change when you drop it on to starchy food, but the paler dilute solution will make it slightly easier to see that it doesn't change when you drop it on to non-starch food. You can test dark liquids or sauces by pouring the tiniest amount of the food – just a mere coating – on to a white saucer. You need very little of the suspect food to test with iodine. You can even dilute food with water if necessary – such as Marmite. The starch will still show up in the food, even if it is quite dilute.

Some foods take longer than others to show the starch content. On nutmeg, for instance, it takes about thirty minutes before the iodine drop turns almost black.

It's surprising to discover that some foods which most people believe to be basically protein – such as certain varieties of nuts – contain high quantities of starch. Ground blanched almonds had never caused me problems, so I wasn't surprised when the iodine test showed they contained no starch. But when I tested them unblanched, they had starch in their skins. The same is true of walnuts. But cashew nuts are very rich in starch, as are chestnuts and sunflower seeds. Peanuts also contain a lot of starch. (Peanuts are not really nuts – they're grown in the earth and are legumes.) Sadly, some of the foods we think of as 'health foods' have high starch content.

Dairy foods do not contain starch, unless it is added or develops naturally, as in the crusts of cheeses such as Brie and Camembert, which may be sprayed with *Penicillium candidum* to produce a mould flora. If you test a little of the crust you'll find it goes quite black, so I would advise cutting these delicious crusts off before eating the cheese.

As I have already mentioned, I am now unable to eat large amounts of dairy foods due to the lactose content. But there's no way of testing for this with the iodine test, which shows only the presence of starch.

Find out what goes into your food

Life becomes much easier when you know a little about cooking. If you've never been much of a cook, now is the time to learn how to identify the ingredients of the food you eat and understand how it is cooked. Unless you know what's in that delicious red-wine sauce on the steak, you're taking a risk every time you order it in a restaurant. The steak itself is starch-free, but the sauce could be cooked either with or without starch. If the chef is using traditional French methods of cooking, he will have used butter or cream to deglaze the sauce (just another word for thickening), and you'll be able to eat it. He may, however, be thickening the sauce with cornflour.

When I first began this diet, I used to hate asking the waiter to find out if there was any flour or cornflour in the sauce. But things have changed. All restaurants are aware of problems with nut allergies and coeliac disease, and because they're so frightened of being sued by customers, they are very scrupulous about telling you exactly what is in the food. Don't be afraid to ask.

You will have to be selective in choosing from the menu. I'm afraid that those pasta, rice and lentil dishes are out, and meat cooked with vegetables, such as casseroles and cassoulets, is dangerous. The chapter on how to eat out will give you more specific help. But there's usually something on a restaurant menu we can eat – even if it's as unadventurous as steak and salad. Just make sure there are no croutons in the salad!

Learn to recognise food additives

As we've already shown in the list of modified starches in Chapter 7, there may be food additives that contain starch in the food you want to eat. I recommend that you buy a copy of the book *E for Additives: The Complete E Number Guide* by Maurice Hanssen.

Most food additives identified by E numbers appear gruesomely suspicious and get a bad press. However, when you look them up in the E-number book, you'll be relieved to find that far from being the dreaded 'man-made chemicals', most are derived from perfectly wholesome plants such as seaweed, or from natural mineral sources which are safe to eat. But sometimes one comes across a food additive that is known to cause digestive problems, and this usually means it will cause problems for people who can't eat starch. The E-number book lists all sources of food additives, which foods they are likely to be added to, and all known adverse effects.

9

How to manage the IBS Low-Starch Diet

Give yourself a reasonable length of time to find out if your symptoms improve. George McCaffery, the first AS sufferer I came in contact with, had amazing relief from symptoms within three days. One AS sufferer, who discovered my first book (written for people with IBS) on the Internet and has now been free of pain for fifteen months on the diet, advises that you stay on the diet for at least a month before giving up. Professor Ebringer recommends at least three months' trial. However, if IBS is your worst problem, you should experience relief from pain and bloating within a shorter time – even days.

You probably think at this stage that you will feel miserable, giving up bread, cakes, pastries and pasta. But keep in mind that what you're giving up is pain! Begin the diet with a positive attitude. What's a few months of not eating these foods? Nothing, in the course of a lifetime. And if at the end of your planned time you don't feel any relief from pain and symptoms, then you can go back to your original diet. But if you experience definite relief from pain, as I did, you'll find it easy to stay on the diet. Life without these symptoms is so wonderful I no longer miss the foods that caused them.

- Read the previous chapter carefully and make sure you have a bottle of iodine and an eyedropper ready to test any food you're unsure about.
- Read the list of ingredients on every can and pack of processed food. (Don't forget to take your reading glasses when you go shopping!) Look out particularly for that little monster 'modified starch'.
- Don't be downhearted if you make mistakes and feel the return of your symptoms – it's not the end of the world. Just start again, knowing that now you can overcome the problem.

Find out which starch, and which *level* of starch, is right for you

The goal of the diet is to find out which and how much starch you need to eliminate to maintain a pain-free, symptom-free life. Not everyone needs to eliminate all starch. One AS sufferer who has had tremendous success on the diet tells me he began with a strict no-starch diet for five months, eating only meat, fish, vegetables, salads and fruit. Now he has been able to introduce bread to his diet in normal quantities. He still can't eat pasta, potatoes and rice.

When I began the diet I eliminated all the grain starches first. For a long time I could eat potatoes and rice. Eventually I had to give these up, but then I do experience the IBS and AS symptoms very severely and need a higher level of starch elimination.

Many people are able to eat a small amount of starch without any problems. You may not need to eliminate all of these foods, especially if you begin the diet early in life. It's a matter of trial and error.

Start slowly: eliminate the most common offenders first

Section 1

Grains, cereals and roots   Anything made with, thickened with or mixed with: arrowroot, baking powder (usually contains wheat flour), barley, barley flour, pearl barley, bran, burghul, bulgur, cornflour, cornmeal, couscous, kazu, matzoh meal, maize flour, malt, malt extract, maize starch, modified starch, oats, oatmeal, polenta, rye, rye flour, sago, semolina, sorghum, tapioca, cracked wheat, wheat flour, wholemeal flour, wheat-germ.

This includes: bread, rolls, buns, croissants, breakfast cereals, muesli, cakes, biscuits, cookies, crackers, pastries, cream puffs, eclairs, pies, flans, quiches, pizzas, battered deep-fried foods, all pasta including canned spaghetti, Italian noodles, egg noodles, wheat noodles, dumplings, doughnuts, pancakes, steamed puddings, batter puddings, bread puddings, crumble-topped puddings, soufflés, custard-powder custards, white sauces, cheese sauce, gravies, sausages, meatloaf, rissoles or any meatballs and mixtures containing breadcrumbs, rusk or modified starch, sandwiches, most pâtés and relishes and chutney, pills and medication in pill form containing maize starch, modified starch or cornflour. Some people may be able to tolerate cornflour when used in small amounts, in, say, Chinese cooking.

Lentils and pulses   Anything made with, thickened with or mixed with: soya beans or soy flour, black fermented Chinese beans, haricot beans, Boston beans, kidney beans, lima beans, pinto beans, broad beans, mung beans, dhal, flageolets, gungo beans, pigeon beans, black-eyed beans, aduki beans, black beans, butter beans, Urd beans, chick beans, cannellini beans, borlotti beans, ful medames, rice beans, lablab beans, red, yellow, brown, grey, orange or green lentils, puy lentils, Indian brown lentils, split peas, chick peas, pigeon peas.

This includes: baked beans, bean salads, soups, casseroles, cassoulets, soya meat substitute, TVP (textured vegetable protein) in loaves, rissoles or patties, bean sauces, soya bean sauce, tamari sauce, pease pudding, shoyu sauce, fu juk.

Soya bean curd (tofu) is a vegetable protein made from soya milk. According to my testing, it contains very little starch. It therefore would be a good source of protein for vegetarians. I have not eaten it myself, but I think it could be eaten on a low-starch diet. If you find that symptoms remain, you will have to eliminate it. Quorn is another protein substitute, a myco-protein product made from a plant similar to mushrooms. It is not high in starch but when tested with iodine it shows the presence of too much starch for me. Some people may be able to eat it.

If symptoms remain or begin to recur, eliminate the second group

Section 2

Rice products   Anything made with, thickened with or mixed with: pudding rice, long-grain rice, brown rice, wild rice, basmati rice, converted rice, easy-cook rice, American rice, Uncle Ben's rice, Italian rice, Carolina rice, glutinous rice, rice noodles.

This includes: rice pudding, rice salads, fried rice, rice served with Indian, Chinese, Italian or Russian dishes, rice noodles, rice paper, stuffings made with rice, rice cakes, Rice Krispies, savoury rice snacks, sweet rice snacks.

Boiled rice, well drained, is less starchy than rice cooked in other ways. Some people may be able to eat it without symptoms returning.

Potato products   Anything made with, thickened with or mixed with: potatoes, potato flour, sweet potatoes, yams.

This includes: potatoes boiled, baked, roasted, scalloped, steamed, fried, battered, deep-fried, candied, chipped, instant potato powder, potato waffles, potato croquettes, crisps, potato salad, potato scones, gnocchi, potato-thickened soups, stews and casseroles – and all the many pre-prepared potato dishes, with or without other vegetables, which you now find on supermarket shelves and in chilled and frozen-food cabinets.

I was able to eat potatoes for two years after having given up grain foods. Some people may be able to include them in their diet permanently.

If symptoms remain or begin to recur, eliminate the third group

Section 3

Cooked fresh vegetables (hot or cold)   Anything cooked with, thickened with or mixed with:

- Root vegetables: parsnips, carrots, celeriac, horseradish, beetroot, breadfruit, taro, cassava, white radish, Chinese radish, Daikon radish, navette, salsify, scorzonera.
- Pods and seeds: green peas, petits pois, mangetout, sugar snap peas, sweetcorn, broad beans, green beans, string beans, flat beans, runner beans, okra.
- Greens: Savoy cabbage, January king cabbage, red cabbage, white cabbage, broccoli, calabrese, cauliflower, Brussels sprouts, spring greens, kale, pak-choi, pe-tsai, kohlrabi.
- Squashes and gourds: pumpkin, butternut squash, spaghetti squash, custard squash, golden nugget, acorn squash, West Indian pumpkin, snake squash, marrow.
- 'Vegetable fruits': aubergines, chilli peppers, akee, breadfruit.

These include: any of the above cooked or canned or bottled, hot or cold, which have been boiled, roasted, baked, scalloped, fried, battered, deep-fried, stir-fried, sautéed, creamed, braised, steamed or grilled, in casseroles, stews, soups, pies, flans, quiches, sauces, pastas, pizzas, curries or salads.

Some people may be able to eat many of these vegetables cooked lightly, in Chinese food and stir-fries, for example. But remember, Chinese cooking almost always contains cornflour and soy sauce. Too much starch for me.

Spices   I have found all spices to contain starch. All peppercorns, whatever their colour, contain starch.

I have not included spices in any of the recipes. But because spices are not used in huge quantities, some people may be able to tolerate the small amount of starch without any problems. You need to experiment for yourself. Small amounts of ground pepper may not cause problems for most people.

10

Is the IBS Low-Starch Diet nutritionally safe?

Chapter 5 has dealt with the nutritional problems of a diet that is too high in starch. But this still doesn't answer the question of whether a diet very low in starch is safe.

No doubt your doctor and your family will be concerned about a diet that seems so unbalanced. But you must remember, you are not eating a diet which contains no carbohydrates – you are simply eliminating the starch part of the carbohydrates.

To repeat what I said in Chapter 5 about carbohydrates, the ideal amount of carbohydrate in an average diet – perfect for keeping the body in great condition – is from 50 to 100gms daily, depending on the individual. But this doesn't have to be in the form of starch. The low-starch diet will give you sufficient carbohydrates in wine, beer, ice-cream, low-starch vegetables and fruit, desserts and cakes.

But one of the objections you may still get from your doctor is about lack of fibre. This is an immediate reaction of doctors and dietitians to a diet that eliminates all grain fibre. But it's wrong. You will be eating fibre in the form of raw fruit and vegetables, and it is increasingly being understood that this is a far better form of fibre. To reassure yourself that the diet is not only delicious but also good for you, spend a few moments reading the following pages.

Is there enough fibre in the IBS Low-Starch Diet?

'Fibre' has become the buzz-word of the nutritional world. Everyone is encouraged to eat more of it to be healthy. Unfortunately, most people (including some doctors and dietitians) seem to have the impression that fibre is found only in wholegrains and bran – all those TV adverts showing plates laden with 'healthy-eating' breakfast cereals have been very persuasive!

For years the standard treatment for IBS has been to put the patient on a high-fibre diet, which has usually meant primarily wholegrains and bran. The results have been dismal. I don't know how many tonnes of bran and wholegrains I have munched through, clutching my stomach in agony at the same time.

We certainly need fibre – most of us have such sluggish guts that we need all the help we can get. We need fibre to provide the bulk that helps push everything through the bowel and to retain the necessary water that keeps stools soft, preventing the hard stools that result in constipation. But wholegrains are not the whole answer.

Bran is the outside skin of wholegrains. The most commonly extracted bran is from wheat. There are a number of disadvantages of bran – both of eating it after extraction and of eating it on the wholegrain or in wholemeal bread. Here are three:

- Bran contains a substance called phytic acid, which is a naturally occurring mineral antagonist in food. This means it interferes with the absorption and utilisation of calcium, magnesium, iron, zinc, copper and vitamin B6 – all of which you need daily.
- Because it is the outside skin of the grain, bran contains a high percentage of the chemicals sprayed on the crop – chemicals that we can't wash off at home. And none of us wants to eat more of those than we have to.
- Researchers studying allergies (allergists) have known for some time about lectins, which are the carbohydrate-binding proteins in most plants. Lectins have numerous effects on our body's cells and tissues, and some are toxic. They cause various conditions in some people, ranging from allergic responses to more serious diseases. For example, lectins are contained in grass and other pollens, and trigger the well-known allergic reactions to these plants in some people. The lectin-rich part of the plant is the skin, and the food that contains the highest rate of lectins is wheatgerm.

Here is a quote from Dr David L.J. Freed, who is one of the contributors to the book *Food Allergy and Intolerance* (Saunders, 2002):

> . . . *wheat lectin (WGA) stands head and shoulders above all others . . . Curious coincidence, then, that wheat is the basic daily staple for most of the Western world, and that wheat is one of the commonest foods responsible for intolerance/allergy. (But rice and maize eaters have no cause to be smug; all cereals have lectins and they are, not surprisingly, very similar.)*

The more I read about wheat, the more I discover that it is the major culprit in many chronic diseases. Doctors and dietitians should no longer be recommending that we eat wholegrains, wheatgerm and bran fibre. Fruit and vegetables contain fibre, and it is becoming more and more obvious that fruit and vegetable fibre is by far the best dietary fibre, whether you're an IBS/AS sufferer or not. Fruit and vegetable fibre also provides you with large quantities of vitamins A, B, C and E, magnesium and a wide range of other minerals.

However, peas, lentils, peanuts, kidney beans, maize, rice, carrots, tomatoes, potatoes, castor oil seeds, soya beans and some edible mushrooms also contain high amounts of lectins. And since we all eat lectins, why don't we all get ill?

Research is continuing on this subject, but it is thought that people who experience the ill effects of lectins do so after they have had a bacterial infection or a bout of influenza. And there are many accounts of IBS or AS being experienced for the first time after these types of illnesses.

But we can all minimise our consumption of lectins. Dr Freed advises:

> *Since vegetable peels and fibres are, by and large, the lectin-rich part of the plant (and also the alkaloid-rich part), I am not therefore altogether happy with the modern trend to 'whole-foods', especially the eating of raw unpeeled vegetables, and I warn my patients to be very careful when patronising 'health food' establishments, as in my view these pose a serious hazard to the health. It is a sad fact that Heaven, for its own inscrutable reasons, has seen fit to make the most nutritious plant foods also the most toxic.*

If someone in your family suffers from mysterious allergies (without symptoms of IBS/AS), it could be due to lectins. Vegetarians are prone to these problems. But they can be overcome by a change of diet which would include reducing wholegrain, bean and lentil intake, and peeling vegetables such as potatoes before cooking and any raw vegetables and fruit before eating.

Salads are delicious and good for you

On the IBS Low-Starch Diet we won't be eating most of the grains and vegetables that are highest in lectins, apart from perhaps tomatoes and mushrooms. As most plants contain lectins, we can't avoid eating them altogether, but we can avoid eating most of them, by peeling our fruit and vegetables.

Most of the vegetables we eat will be raw. This is because although most raw vegetables contain starch, when they are eaten raw, the starch passes through the digestive system, sealed in the vegetable cell. The digestive juices cannot easily penetrate this vegetable cell, which is rather like a waterproof envelope. When vegetables are cooked the vegetable cell is broken down, and this is when the starch is released, causing symptoms of IBS and AS.

Vitamins are lost when vegetables are cooked

One of the major disadvantages of cooking vegetables (except for those which cannot be eaten raw, such as potatoes and lentils) is that much of their important vitamin content is lost during cooking, either because the vitamins are destroyed by heat or because they are lost in the cooking water. These are known as the water-soluble vitamins. All are needed by your body every day, but your body is unable to store them longer than a day at a time, because any left over from your daily needs are excreted in your urine. For this reason you need to eat them every day.

Green leafy vegetables, tomatoes and fruit contain small amounts of vitamins B1 and B2, and larger amounts of another B vitamin, niacin, all of which are in danger of being lost in cooking. They are also a major source of one of the most important water-soluble vitamins – ascorbic acid, or vitamin C.

On the IBS Low-Starch Diet you'll be eating salads almost every day and will be getting good supplies of vitamin C daily.

A further word from Dr Freed:

Allergists who use the 'Stone-age Diet' [the IBS Low-Starch Diet is a good example], *which eliminates most carbohydrate foods and therefore most lectins, report that this diet appears to confer a large degree of immunity to common upper respiratory infections. Many patients (and I myself) notice that they only catch colds if they were 'cheating' at the time of virus exposure, by eating bread or some other forbidden luxury . . .*

Which brings me to . . .

The importance of proteins

At the risk of being repetitive (but I know that many people 'chapter hop' and miss out on important information) I will once again talk about the need for protein in our diets. Protein foods are the most important part of everyone's dietary needs. Although the IBS Low-

Starch Diet eliminates so many starch foods, it is rich in protein. The main sources of protein are (in descending order):

- eggs
- milk and milk products
- liver and other glandular meats
- muscle meats
- fish and fowl
- yeast
- wheatgerm
- soya flour
- some nuts

On the IBS Low-Starch Diet we will not be eating any yeast, wheatgerm, soya flour or most nuts apart from almonds, because although these are plant proteins, they also contain starch. However, plant proteins are not 'complete' proteins – in other words, they lack some of the essential amino acids. Therefore they are of value as proteins *only* when eaten with eggs, milk or meat, or with the correct complementary combination of other plant proteins (not easy!), to ensure that all the essential amino acids are provided in the diet. This is why, in a normal diet, breakfast cereals are eaten with milk, toast is buttered, cakes are made with eggs/butter/milk, and so on.

Most people in Western countries should be able to get sufficient protein from a normal, well-balanced diet. However, people recovering from illnesses or going on a weight-loss diet should increase their protein intake.

But if you're trying to lose weight, there's another very interesting reason why you should specifically eliminate wheat products from your diet.

One final word from Dr Freed:

> *It has been known for over twenty years that WGA* [wheat lectin] *and many other lectins act on adipocytes* [fat cells] *and other tissue cells just like insulin in terms of anabolism* [the building of body tissues], *cell proliferation, lipogenesis* [fat formation], *and anti-lipolysis* [prevention of fat being broken down in the body]. *This is the insulinomimetic effect . . . and possibly sheds new light on why wheat makes people fat.*

If your diet until now has been a low-protein diet, consisting mainly of bread, cereals, pasta and foods made from wheat, the IBS Low-Starch

Diet will not only eliminate your painful symptoms, but also boost your energy levels and feelings of well-being – and help you achieve your ideal weight.

But what about the cholesterol monster?

The IBS Low-Starch Diet has definite advantages for people worried about cholesterol levels.

- Your intake of fatty foods will be dramatically lowered, because you won't be eating buttered bread, toast, rolls, scones, buns, or deep-fried fast foods such as fish and chips, or snack foods such as crisps. You also won't be eating all the high-starch cakes and pastries made with butter or margarine (and many margarines are cholesterol culprits). Although the IBS Low-Starch Diet gives recipes for puddings and desserts made with cream and dairy products, they are made with ground almonds, which is richer than flour, and you will find you can't eat as much because you are satisfied more quickly.

- You will find that your desire for sweet, fatty foods gradually diminishes on the IBS Low-Starch Diet. This is because when you are eating a diet adequate in protein, your hunger is satisfied for longer and you don't have the dramatic dips in blood sugar levels that make you crave sweet foods.

- It is now known that fruit and vegetable fibre is better than bran or grain fibre at lowering blood cholesterol levels. Higher consumption of fruit and vegetables is associated with a lower risk of coronary heart disease.

What if you're vegetarian?

Believe it or not, I would love to have been able to be a vegetarian. Vegetables are by far my favourite foods. I have every sympathy for people who have been vegetarian most of their lives and can't face the thought of eating meat. But the IBS Low-Starch Diet is extremely difficult for people who don't eat some meat or fish. A vegetarian diet is usually full of bread and grain products, and it's difficult enough for vegetarians at the best of times to keep up their protein levels without cutting out beans and lentils – foods which are, unfortunately, among the highest in starch.

If you feel from the symptoms I've described that eliminating starch would help you, you will have to eat large amounts of fruit and raw vegetables and a serving of cheese or eggs at every meal.

However, vegans will find it almost impossible to get enough of the right foods to sustain good health. Tofu (bean curd) is worth trying as it contains only small amounts of starch. Quorn and TVP are too starchy for me but some people may be able to eat them without experiencing symptoms. However, many foods made from these products seem to be coated in bread-crumbs or have flour added, which greatly increases the starch content.

If you are experiencing IBS/AS badly, I would recommend a week's trial of the first stage of the IBS Low-Starch Diet, and if you experience relief from symptoms, no matter how slight, then you may be able to work out a satisfactory diet without bread and lentils, but it will not be easy.

11

What can I eat?

Now for the good news – and there's plenty of it, despite the huge list of things we can't eat. The IBS Low-Starch Diet is not another dreary, tasteless, 'lettuce leaf and nut cutlet' regime. Many of our recipes are very sophisticated – even decadent. You might discover that food has never tasted better.

All-protein foods

- Beef, lamb, pork, poultry and game, roasted, grilled, boiled, baked, poached, scalloped, casseroled, stewed and braised. These can be seasoned with herbs, mustard, wine, honey, dried onion or garlic, fruits (fresh or dried). Sauces and gravies can be thickened with mustard, butter, cream, crème fraîche and yoghurt.
- All cooked whole meats and fish, such as ham, pastrami, corned beef, chicken, turkey, bacon, smoked salmon and other smoked fish.
- All starch-free processed meat, poultry and fish products, such as European sausages, pepperoni, salami, liver sausage and some pâtés.
- All fresh, frozen and canned fish such as salmon, tuna, herrings, sardines, kippers, unless in a sauce containing starch. (No battered or breadcrumb-coated fish.)

Fruit and vegetables

- All fruits, raw and cooked, except bananas – with the recommendation that because of modern supermarket storing methods you test for starch before eating. (Two other fruits which I cannot be sure of are mangos and pineapples. When I tested these and found them to contain starch, they were imported fruits and may have been picked green and cold-stored, so that the starch did not turn to fructose. If naturally ripened, they may be safe to eat. Test avocado before eating as this is often cold-stored).

- All canned fruits with the possible exception of mangos and pineapple.
- All raw salad vegetables: lettuce, spinach, celery, herbs, tomatoes, peppers, cucumber, fennel, onions, spring onions, mushrooms, peppers (red, yellow and orange are best. Green peppers are really unripened).
- Cooked vegetables: asparagus, spinach, fennel, tomatoes, mushrooms, peppers and garlic (in moderation. I include garlic in cooking for flavour and do not usually eat the bulb). Onions, shallots and leeks do not contain starch and can be eaten raw or cooked, but some people may find that cooked in certain ways they cause indigestion. The caramelisation (browning) of onions when fried, for example, often causes problems even for normal people because it produces digestive-resistant starch.

Herbs, spices, jams, sauces and condiments

- All herbs, dried and fresh.
- Salt.
- Mustard made *without* wheat flour is completely safe. These are usually German or French mustards. (Check the labels.) Other spices are to be used with caution.
- Dried garlic powder and onion powder.
- Cocoa (which is a berry) may be eaten or drunk in moderation.
- Honey, maple syrup, golden syrup, all jams and jellies that are not thickened with starch.

Dairy foods

Eat and drink as many varieties of dairy foods as you can. This includes milk, cream, cheese, yoghurt and all the variations of these foods. However, milk contains lactose, a disaccharide which causes IBS symptoms in some people (this is known as lactose intolerance). When milk is correctly digested, the lactose is broken down into glucose and galactose. But if you can't digest it properly, then it ferments in the gut causing pain, bloating and diarrhoea. Refer to Chapter 7 for further information on how you might be able to overcome these symptoms, and look for lactose-free recipes throughout.

Sweets and desserts

Ice-cream, mousse, sorbet, fruit yoghurt, egg custard, crème brûlée, crème caramel, custard sauces, meringues, fruit sauces, toffees, fudge, chocolates, cakes and biscuits made with ground almonds. Jellies including fresh fruit and/or alcohol, or made with flavoured gelatine or pectin.

Beverages

The cup that cheers and all the other cheery drinks can be part of the IBS Low-Starch Diet. This includes tea, coffee, wine, spirits, beer, cider and lager. Although whisky, bourbon and vodka are distilled from grains and/or potatoes, the distilling process removes the starch. I haven't tested every brand on the market! If you're worried, test a small amount before you drink.

Most soft drinks are starch-free, but beware of lemon barley water which, if made correctly, contains barley flour. Some brands of bitter lemon now have starch added. You should also be cautious about malted milk shakes and milk drinks which contain malt extract. Test before drinking.

I have discovered that orange juice in cardboard packs often contains starch. Most paper and cardboard (except coffee filters) contains a great deal of starch, and it may be that in the case of orange juice, the acid in the juice permeates the wax lining, allowing small amounts of starch to come through. However, because the pith of the orange contains starch, it could also be that starch is released in the pressing of the fruit. Milk does not appear to be affected by the cardboard cartons.

This may not affect you unless you are particularly sensitive, but in recent years I have tended to be cautious about fruit juices, simply because of modern storage methods for fruit. I would advise you to test before drinking a new brand.

Fruit juices and hot drinks used to be painful for me to drink before I eliminated starch. I have come to the conclusion that my digestive tract was so aggravated before I eliminated starch that acidic and hot drinks caused pain. Now it is blissfully calm. I also now do not suffer from reflux problems and indigestion after meals.

Medicines

Most tablets and pills contain starch and cannot be included in the IBS Low-Starch Diet without causing symptoms. It will probably be quite frightening to contemplate giving up the very medicines you feel are the only things keeping you going. These will often be pain-relievers, such as paracetamol or aspirin-based medications, and perhaps tranquillisers.

You may, however, find that the medication you are taking is available in liquid or starch-free formulation. For example, I take a diuretic which my GP prescribes in liquid form.

If you are taking any tranquillisers, it is *essential* that you consult your doctor before trying to give up.

Pain-relievers

These are available in liquid or starch-free forms. Ask your doctor to prescribe them, or buy Aspro-clear or Alka-seltzer from your chemist or supermarket. (Alka-seltzer is an excellent pain-reliever and contains aspirin but also sodium bicarbonate, which makes it very easy on the stomach.)

Alternative medicines

An increasing number of starch and gluten-free vitamin supplements and herbal remedies are now on the market. Check the labels before buying. Homeopathic pills contain only minute amounts of starch and you may be able to continue taking these. (I understand that liquid versions of homeopathic remedies are available through homeopathic practitioners.)

Laxatives

If you regularly take laxatives, Epsom salts (which I take on the advice of a specialist at St Mark's Hospital, London) contain no starch and are excellent and non-habit-forming. I take between 1½ and 2 teaspoons every night, dissolved in a glass of water. Drink it down quickly. It tastes horrible, but it really works and doesn't make you feel ill, like other laxatives.

Epsom salts is an old-fashioned remedy which lost favour when new, 'improved' drugs and herbal pills became available. Most of these, however, have proved habit-forming and many doctors are now returning to Epsom salts.

The correct chemical name for Epsom salts is magnesium sulphate. Magnesium is one of the minerals essential for good health. If you want to reassure yourself about this much-neglected mineral – which has many other health-promoting properties, including helping to relieve premenstrual tension, muscle cramps and fatigue and lowering high blood pressure in women – refer to *Nutritional Medicine* by Dr Stephen Davies and Dr Alan Stewart (Pan Books, 1987). Magnesium is also available as Milk of Magnesia and as various magnesium tablets. Just make sure they're starch-free.

Examples from my daily diet

These are the sort of things I eat every day, whether at home or out. The IBS Low-Starch Diet doesn't allow for lazy shopping – you have to have more in the cupboard than a loaf of bread and a pack of butter. Basically, from now on, you'll be living on a hunter-gatherer's diet, or 'Stone-Age' diet, as it is sometimes called, and you'll have to make sure you do plenty of hunting and gathering of the right foods.

At every meal I make sure I have both carbohydrate and protein. Protein keeps you going far longer than carbohydrate. If you don't believe that, just see what happens when you eat bacon and eggs for breakfast instead of the usual bowl of cereal. The carbohydrate you eat will be in the form of raw vegetables and/or the limited selection of cooked vegetables, fruit both dried and fresh, cooked or uncooked, a selection of syrups and spreads, selected sweets and desserts, and the cakes, cookies and puddings from the recipe section.

Breakfast is the meal that causes most problems to most people. Before you began this diet you were probably used to having just a bowl of cereal or a couple of pieces of toast. Or even worse, perhaps you skipped breakfast. If you take the time to have a good breakfast you will be amazed at how it makes you smarter and more energetic throughout the day. A good breakfast will stop you longing for those starchy goodies mid-morning that always make you feel bloated and tired. Even if you don't feel you can face more than coffee or tea first thing, make sure you have something to eat with it. It will take away that depressed, anxious feeling that makes mornings so miserable.

Breakfast

Cooked fruit such as prunes or other cooked or canned fruit. Fresh fruit such as melon (or any starch-free fruit). Starch-free yoghurt. Fresh, frozen or smoked fish. Eggs scrambled, fried, poached or boiled. Bacon, starch-free sausages, salami, ham. Maple syrup. Coffee, tea, etc.

I usually begin with smoked salmon and a slice or two of melon with my early-morning coffee. Now, I know this sounds incredibly indulgent, but I don't have a huge serving of either, and they both last for several days, in the fridge. The reason I eat them together is that they give me both protein and carbohydrate and they're not too heavy for first thing. You *could* simply have that before you set off to work – they're almost as instant as a bowl of cereal.

However, my usual routine is then to shower and dress before eating a proper breakfast: two rashers of grilled bacon with maple syrup and two fried or scrambled eggs. I discovered, while on holiday in America, how good maple syrup tastes on bacon. Everyone else was having bacon and pancakes with maple syrup, but I just poured it on my bacon and eggs. After all, scrambled eggs are just pancakes with the flour left out! And maple syrup is a starch-free carbohydrate which helps to keep up your carb consumption. This breakfast will never make you feel full, but it's amazingly sustaining and keeps me going so well that I can often skip lunch, although by teatime I usually need a snack.

Lunch

Cheese, ham, pastrami, salmon, tuna, left-over cold chicken from last night's supper or cottage cheese with salad or an apple. Simple hot dishes such as Bacon Star or Creamy Salmon Bake (see index) or an omelette. McDonald's cheeseburgers (without the bun) and salad. Yoghurt, cooked or raw fresh or dried fruit, ice-cream, meringue, cake or biscuits made from ground almonds, coffee, tea or soft drink.

If you're at work you won't be able to simply grab a sandwich. You could take your lunch to work with you, but if not you'll have to find a café or restaurant where you can get a salad with meat, eggs or fish. There's usually no problem in a restaurant, and I find that even coffee bars or sandwich bars where they make up your sandwich of choice are happy to give me a plate of ham with salad. If you're longing for something sweet, order a vanilla ice-cream and an espresso coffee. Pour the espresso over the ice-cream. Delicious!

Dinner

Meat, chicken or fish, braised, roasted, fried, grilled or casseroled with dried onion, dried or fresh garlic, herbs, tomatoes, wine, mustard, lemon juice, dried or fresh fruit. Mixed salad and/or cooked spinach, asparagus, fennel, mushrooms or tomatoes. Ice-cream, sorbet, yoghurt, mousse, jelly, chocolates, meringues, egg custard, crème brûlée, crème caramel, cakes, biscuits or desserts made with ground almonds, cooked or canned fruit or fresh fruit salad with cream.

The foods you will now have to eliminate are, of course, all the exotic dishes that have become so much part of our diet these days: Italian pastas, Indian curries, oriental rice dishes, as well as the many and varied potato and vegetarian dishes that are out there. But you can still serve these up for your family while you eat your chicken or steak and salad, or you can give them the same as you are eating, with additional servings of starchy foods and vegetables. In the recipe section I tell you how to cook a roast without cooking the potatoes in the same pan as the meat, and how to make gravy without flour or granules.

Snacks

Cold meats, pâté with tomato, pepperoni, dried fruit such as raisins, salted toasted almonds, dates, apricots, peaches, cheese, yoghurt, cakes and biscuits made with ground almonds, ice-cream, ice-lollies, chocolate or non-starch sweets. (Dates with cream cheese or slices of cheese wrapped in lettuce make great snacks.)

Don't let yourself get hungry. Make sure you have supplies of snacking food on hand. There are so many single-serving ice-creams and ice-lollies available – just make sure they don't contain starch. And dried fruit these days is anything but dry. There are wonderful soft and succulent sweetened dried fruits available – try peaches and apricots.

Drinks

Neither coffee nor tea is a problem. I usually drink coffee for breakfast only, but I drink two strong cups, and now that I've given up dairy foods I use Coffeemate. Many people worry about caffeine, and I used to think coffee gave me indigestion, but when I gave up starch I never had indigestion again.

During the day I drink water and the occasional soft drink such as Coca-Cola. I would prefer to drink fruit juice, but I never know without testing whether it has been made from unripened fruit and will have too much starch for me. Soft drinks such as Coca-Cola never cause me any problems, and the sugar (I don't like diet drinks) gives me an energy burst.

I enjoy the occasional gin and tonic, and wine with my evening meal.

12

The side effects of a low-starch diet

First the good news

One of the surprising and welcome side effects I have noticed is that I now rarely feel the cold. As a child I used to suffer from bad circulation in cold weather – my music teacher always had to give me five minutes of hand exercises before I could begin to play the piano. Chilblains were agony every winter. Even as an adult, I once developed the early stages of gangrene in one of my toes because of lack of blood. Now I notice that I feel quite warm when others around me are huddled into thick clothes, complaining of feeling chilly. Perhaps I've discovered the secret of the Eskimos' ability to withstand the cold.

Another inevitable side effect is that you will lose weight. After years of yo-yo dieting, my weight now never deviates. I can wear the same clothes for years (not always an advantage!). I have had letters from readers who say that after trying every diet on the market without success (they've even *gained* weight on low-fat diets), within weeks of beginning the IBS Low-Starch Diet, they have lost weight, and kept it off for the first time in their lives.

And they all say they have never had such energy. I certainly agree with this. Of course, simply eliminating the exhausting symptoms of pain makes a huge difference to your energy reserves. But I have noticed how much more energy I have than other healthy people of my age. I run upstairs, two at a time. It never occurs to me to need a midday snooze.

Now the bad news

One disadvantage of the IBS Low-Starch Diet (apart from the obvious ones!) is connected with the fact that starch is the 'tranquilliser' of the food world. A large piece of cake is definitely soothing. That's why so many people are driven to binge on packets of chocolate biscuits and other sweet foods when they're upset. Experts call this 'carbohydrate craving'. I prefer to call it starch addiction, because it is the starch rather than the carbohydrate that causes the craving. All of these foods that are so soothing and that you can binge on so easily are 'refined carbohydrates' – in other words, starch. The carbohydrate part has been virtually eliminated.

If you continue to stuff yourself with too many starchy foods, your body becomes physically addicted to them. The more starch you eat, the more insulin the body must produce in order to digest it. The body produces insulin in order to convert into glucose the sugar that has accumulated in your blood from the starch you've just eaten. The more insulin your body releases – the more quickly it converts the sugar into glucose – the quicker your blood sugar levels will drop, making you crave those starches again. Starch addiction is a vicious circle which requires the production of ever more and more insulin, until ultimately your body rebels and develops a condition known as insulin resistance, which can lead to diabetes mellitus.

When you first begin the diet and your body is unused to going without starch, you may find that you behave like a hungry baby and feel like screaming at people. Babies, of course, do live on a starch-free diet (so that's one way we know that it's not unhealthy!) but are very sensitive to hunger pangs. Be prepared to eat immediately you get that empty feeling. Keep plenty of low-starch snacks available. If you have to binge, binge on protein foods. Protein and fatty foods satisfy your appetite far more thoroughly. You can't eat nearly as much at one sitting, but what you do eat will keep you satisfied for longer.

You will get used to doing without starch in time, especially if you make sure you always have a good breakfast. You have to get into the habit of thinking ahead where meals are concerned. Make sure you take food with you when you're out, or stop and eat even if you don't feel like it, when you get the chance. You may not have the chance in an hour or so, when you will feel hungry.

If you also suffer from hypoglycaemia (low blood sugar)

You will probably already have experienced faintness and confusion when you're hungry – even on a normal diet. Hypoglycaemia is caused by a deficiency of glucose in the bloodstream (all carbohydrates have to be broken down by the digestive system to be turned into glucose). The moment you feel the symptoms of low blood sugar, you need food immediately. If bread and starchy foods make up a large part of your diet, you may find that when you first give them up you will experience headaches, weakness, faintness, even panic attacks. In fact, you may not even have been aware until then that you suffer from hypoglycaemia – it often goes undiagnosed for years.

Because glucose is the sole source of energy for the brain, a deficiency of glucose will cause these symptoms often before you even know you're hungry. Other symptoms can range from irritability, nausea, fast heartbeat, anxiety, cold sweats and even vertigo, to behaviour problems and mood swings.

For many years doctors have been advising patients to eat a quick carbohydrate meal to boost their low blood sugar levels. However, recent medical thinking on this problem has changed. I quote again from *Nutritional Medicine* by Dr Stephen Davies and Dr Alan Stewart:

> *One of the commonest contributing factors in hypoglycaemia in the West is excessive refined carbohydrate consumption . . . Some doctors are under the misconception that if a person has a low blood sugar they should simply have a cup of tea with a few teaspoonfuls of sugar. This is wrong. Whilst this might well produce relief of the symptoms for a while, it encourages a vicious circle; a low blood sugar, refined carbohydrate ingestion, excessive insulin secretion, followed by a low blood sugar. One approach to treatment of low blood sugar is the elimination of refined carbohydrates from the diet.*

Other writers on the subject recommend eating five or six small meals a day that are low in simple carbohydrates, moderate in fats and high in protein, composed of meat, fish, eggs, cheese and vegetables.

One of the greatest difficulties of the IBS Low-Starch Diet is that when you're out, you can't grab a quick sandwich. Read Chapter 13, on eating out, and learn which fast foods are safe.

You must make sure you eat regular, frequent meals – don't wait until you feel hunger pangs. Make cakes, biscuits, candies and sweets from the baking recipes in this book and carry them with you if you're travelling. Take cheese segments, dried or fresh fruit, almonds and sliced meats. I usually make sure I have several small packets of raisins in my bag when I'm travelling. You never know when you're going to be stuck in a traffic jam or delayed on a train.

I also find sweet soft drinks, such as Coke, Pepsi and Fanta, very reviving when I've gone too long without food. Believe it or not, they are better than the healthier alternative of fruit juices – which may contain unripened starch.

13

Guide to eating out

Eating out at someone else's home is very difficult. Despite the fact that so many people nowadays do not eat various foods (which makes catering for a dinner party a nightmare), most of your friends will find cooking a starch-free meal very difficult – they simply don't realise the number of foods that contain starch. It's embarrassing to have to lay down rules in someone else's house. Unless you've been invited to your nearest and dearest's for dinner, you may find it better to confess your problem and bring your own food. I have often taken my own chicken salad rather than inconvenience the hostess. You can always suggest that you arrive after the meal, but if you say (firmly) that the company is more important to you than the food, then your hostess won't feel awkward.

Eating at a party is not quite so problematic – there's sure to be something on the table you can nibble at to stave off hunger pangs. However, many parties these days are 'themed' and you may discover the food is entirely spicy curries or something else that causes you problems. Be prepared not to eat much. I usually eat something at home before I go so that I can last the distance.

Restaurants are easier. Most have some dishes on the menu that can be eaten on the IBS Low-Starch Diet. Grilled meats, poultry, fish (cooked without flour), salad (no cooked vegetables, beans, croutons, etc.), followed by dessert such as ice-cream or sorbet will be fine. If you fancy a meat or fish dish cooked in a sauce, ask the waiter to find out if it contains flour or cornflour. So many people nowadays can't eat wheat flour or have a food allergy that restaurants are aware of the dangers of their customers getting ill. I find waiters are very willing to help.

As I have said throughout the book, everyone must find the level of starch they are most comfortable with. Below is a list of the restaurants I can and can't eat at. But even in restaurants that I would not risk, if you give up the bread rolls, the bread-sticks, the naan bread, chapatis, dishes made with potatoes, lentils and peanuts, you may be able to eat other things on the menu.

Who's out (for me)

Chinese

Rice is definitely out for me, and even stir-fried vegetables are a problem. Chinese cooking also includes lots of soy sauce (soya beans are lentils) and modified starch in the form of cornflour. You may find it doesn't contain too much starch for you, but take note of what your body tells you. I have eaten Chinese food in Taiwan, but it was only asparagus with plain grilled chicken or beef. Everyone else had wonderful dishes that I was too scared to try. I still had a good time!

Indian

Rice is not the only problem here. Despite the fact that properly made curries are not thickened with flour or cornflour (they are mostly yoghurt), there are many ingredients in Indian cooking that are too starchy for me. Ginger, whether fresh or dried, is one of them. Most of the vegetables and spices are also too starchy for me. Many of you may still be able to eat the meat or vegetable curries without the breads. I adore curries. Even the smell is exquisite. It is heartbreaking to have to go without these wonderful dishes, but I keep in mind that it's really only pain I'm going without.

The local chippy

No fish and chips, I'm sad to say! But if the local chippy sells fried chicken, providing it has no batter, I can eat that – without chips.

Who's not recommended

Vegetarian

Unless I eat only salads.

Teashops and coffee bars

These are not easy. Most of the food choices are sandwiches, filled rolls, cakes and pastries. Sometimes I can buy salads or yoghurts (look carefully at the ingredients on the pack). I may have to settle for cheese segments or an ice-cream sundae. I go to all these places with friends if I'm out, but I usually only have a drink. And because I've had a good breakfast, I don't feel hungry.

Who's in

Pizza parlours

Strange as it may seem, I can always eat something at a pizza parlour. On occasions, I have even carefully picked my way through a pizza by eating only the topping. But most pizza restaurants also have salads, so it's safer to stick to those.

Pizza Express have several salads that I have eaten for years without any problems. Their salad dressings are also starch-free.

I also find that pizza restaurants are usually happy to prepare a special dish of something I can eat. They have plenty of supplies of salami and ham in the kitchen and will cheerfully make up a dish of assorted meats with a salad if you explain you have an eating disorder.

Cafés

Fried eggs, poached eggs, scrambled eggs, bacon, grilled tomatoes. I don't eat the sausages or toast.

Pubs

I order a plain steak or a ham or cheese ploughman's. Sometimes I ask what they serve with the ploughman's or say I don't want anything but a plain green salad with tomatoes. Or sometimes I just leave the bread rolls, French fries, pickled onion and chutney. I am always wary of potato salad, coleslaw, beetroot and cooked cold vegetables in the salad.

English restaurants and steakhouses

I find it best to order a plain steak and salad, without French fries, potatoes or any other vegetables, except perhaps asparagus or spinach. If the steak comes with a sauce, I ask whether it is thickened with flour or cornflour. I often ask for mustard (such as Dijon) instead.

French

Order carefully and ask the waiter to help. If the restaurant values its reputation it will be happy to tell you what each dish contains. You may have to order something simple like steak. Remember, the French are very literal about their salads. If you order a green salad you will get just that – lettuce only. If you order a tomato salad, that is all you will get. I always order both. Most cream or wine sauces cooked by French chefs are made without cornflour or flour – see recipe section for the correct methods of making cream and wine sauces. There's sure to be a starch-free dessert on the menu. Otherwise, have a liqueur or glass of sweet wine.

Italian

The best restaurants I have ever eaten at are Italian restaurants in Italy. Despite its reputation for being a nation of pasta eaters, Italy has a most varied national cuisine and produces a huge range of dishes made with the purest, freshest, simplest low-starch ingredients. Look up the Italian for 'I cannot eat bread or flour' and they will shake their heads sadly but, nevertheless, bring you fabulous food.

Spanish

The much-loved paella would be out for me, but the Spanish have many wonderful meat and fish dishes that I am able to eat. Ask your waiter to translate for you.

Greek/Lebanese restaurants

Much Greek and Lebanese food is very simply cooked, without complicated sauces. Their grilled lamb and chicken dishes are wonderful. Greek salads are a meal in themselves. But beware of taramasalata, which contains bread, and hummus, which is made with chickpeas. Many of their sweet dishes are very starchy.

Moroccan/Tunisian

I must confess I've never eaten at these restaurants, but looking at the recipes I can see I would have to be very careful. So many of their dishes are made with lentils of various sorts, which are also added to their vegetable dishes. I would have to avoid all these. However, grilled vegetable salads made with peppers and tomatoes would probably be fine, as would their fresh salads. I would enquire about the ingredients in their meat and fish dishes. These look wonderful and many of them are cooked with fruit and will be free of high-starch ingredients. Ask your waiter to help you.

Japanese grills

These are the most wonderful restaurants for me because they serve steak, fish and many other foods that I can eat, in addition to traditional

Japanese. And because the food is prepared and cooked in front of your eyes, you can see exactly what goes into it. I avoid the traditional Japanese dishes because so many of them come with rice or noodles. Highly recommended.

McDonald's

Fast food is not a new invention. In Victorian times, the streets of London rang with the sounds of fast-food vendors selling their wares. Pies, pasties, muffins, oysters, winkles, jellied eels, watercress were all foods bought and often eaten on the street. Many of the thousands of people who had left the country to find work in the cities lived in tiny rooms without even a kitchen. So in a way, fast food is a time-honoured tradition in Britain. But sadly, fast foods today are usually full of starch.

Well, contrary as it may sound, McDonald's is a life-saver for those of us who can't eat starch. If you've always associated McDonald's with the dreaded description 'junk food', read Chapter 5 for the real truth about junk foods.

If you'd told me years ago that I would gaze with delight on the familiar McDonald's sign I would never have believed you. But when you're tired and hungry, and scared to try unfamiliar food, those golden arches are like a magnet.

McDonald's nutritional analysis of what their hamburgers and other foods contain compares favourably with recommended diets. They are constantly updating their menus to give customers a choice of less fatty foods. And best of all, they don't change the ingredients. This may sound like a gourmet's nightmare, but for those of us who *have* to know what our food contains, you always know exactly what you're getting at McDonald's, regardless of which country you're in. They're not suddenly going to bulk up their burger patties with breadcrumbs or thicken their shakes with modified starch.

All over the world McDonald's hamburgers are made from 100 per cent meat and are safe for us to eat on the IBS Low-Starch Diet. Of course – we can't eat the bun.

I recommend the cheeseburger. It's easily removed from the bun (wear your glasses as you must make sure no little pieces of bread stick to the burger) and the burger is slim enough to fold over and eat with the sticky sauce and cheese inside, like a sandwich. It's not as messy as it sounds, but you do need to have plenty of paper napkins.

I have never had any trouble eating cheeseburgers (without the bun you'll need at least two) and I've never found the gherkin slice to cause me any problems, although this can be easily discarded. The plain hamburger, the quarterpounder and the quarterpounder with cheese are all safe to eat (although the bigger burgers are a little chunky to fold over). The Big Mac sauce, however, contains modified starch, and so does the quarterpounder with cheese deluxe, which includes a mayonnaise with modified starch.

McDonald's thickshakes are made from skimmed milk, cream and various other flavourings and stabilisers, but they contain no starch thickening. Their ice-cream sundaes are also starch-free and so are the sauces, except the fudge sauce. All their beverages (with perhaps the exception of orange juice) are starch-free.

In my opinion, McDonald's reputation for 'junk food' is undeserved. There are many other food manufacturers who would more accurately fit this description. McDonald's are very aware of their reputation and are making efforts to provide a wider range of salads and fresh fruit. These change from country to country, and even from city to city, so I can't give examples here. But I have learned you can count on McDonald's to provide a reliable standard of quality, internationally.

Other fast-food burger chains may have starch-free foods, but I am not aware of many. Burger King's hamburgers, for example, are 100 per cent beef, but their mayonnaise, ketchup and Cheddar cheese fillings contain modified starch. Their milk shakes and ice-creams, however, are free of starch additives.

14

Recipes

- All the recipes are in the very-low-to-no-starch category and can be eaten at any stage of the diet.
- If you are still in the early stages of elimination, add servings of potatoes, rice or cooked vegetables.
- Your family and friends will also enjoy these recipes. Just add servings of pasta, rice, bread, potatoes or cooked vegetables for people with normal health.
- Note: cup measurements are for the British cup = ½ pint = 10 fl oz = 300 ml.

Some changes

Since I wrote my first book I have refined my recipes even further. Some ingredients I thought contained starch – perhaps because I had tested them in an unripened state – I have now discovered do not contain starch if they are properly ripened. Some spices, such as pepper, can no longer be included because I have discovered they do contain remarkable amounts of starch. Fructose or fruit sugar, which I used to use frequently, is not always readily available. I have also come to the conclusion that it doesn't really make a huge difference unless the food is being cooked for several hours, so I have removed it from most of the recipes.

I have also included a number of new lactose-free recipes. Many of you may always have been unable to digest dairy foods, or may discover as you get older that this becomes the case. This happened to me. My lingering, spasmodic AS symptoms disappeared when I gave up dairy foods on a regular basis. The lactose-free recipes are identified throughout.

Low-starch cooking is just as easy as everyday cooking, but there are some new rules. Apart from eliminating the obvious forms of starch as already discussed, many of the processed convenience foods you've used in the past, such as stock cubes or Gravox, Bisto, Marmite and Bovril, should not be used, as they all contain starch of some sort. All vegetable stock cubes also contain starch. Most spices should be avoided, either fresh or raw. Ginger, for example, one of the most delicious additions to spicy foods, is a root and very starchy, even as a powder. Cinnamon, a bark, also contains starch. But there are plenty of ways to 'beef' up the taste of your food – in fact, you'll discover a whole new range of lovely flavours.

Herbs do not contain starch, either raw or cooked, fresh or dried, and I find them a valuable addition to many dishes. Mustard is also starch-free according to the iodine test, and available in so many different flavour variations that you'll find it a great standby. I always have at least three varieties on hand to use in different ways instead of stock cubes.

Start shopping

Pack identification

The first thing to remember when you're buying canned, chilled, frozen or processed foods of any kind is to read the back of the pack – every pack. Become a connoisseur of that list of ingredients. It's surprising where and how often modified starch is used, and regrettably, it's on the increase.

A huge range of foods must, of necessity, contain wheat flour or modified starch and you'll quickly learn which they are. But in many cases, modified starch is entirely unnecessary as a recipe ingredient. It's used simply to make foods cheaper to produce.

Foods to which you would not add thickening if you were making them in your home, such as baby foods, lemon curd, chutneys and pickles, often contain starch when they're commercially prepared. Canned, dried and chilled soups always contain starch of some sort. Even some shop-bought oil and vinegar dressings contain modified starch, even in France, the home of the vinaigrette. Some mayonnaises contain modified starch and some do not. In some ice-creams, the fruit and chocolate fudge sauce or ripples contain modified starch. Some yoghurts do, some don't. Under EU regulations they are not required to say whether they contain starch, and I have discovered that certain brands do add starch even when they state on the label that they are 'low-fat natural yoghurt containing nothing but milk and bacteria'.

Keep these flavour-enhancers in your store cupboard

Dried onions   Onion flakes, which I included in many of the recipes in my first book, seem not to be available now. Dried onion granules and dried minced onion have perhaps replaced them, and are starch-free. Both are an excellent substitute for fresh onions.

I am still undecided as to whether fresh onions are risky in cooking. I know I can eat them raw, but in the past I believed them to be starchy when cooked. This may have been due to the type of onion I tested. I recently tested a wide range of onions, including leeks and shallots, both raw and after cooking, and discovered all except red onions to be negative for starch. However, it has long been known that in certain people onions cause indigestion and flatulence. People who can't eat fresh onions have no trouble with dried.

Dried garlic granules When I wrote my first book I referred to a reference book called *The Composition of Foods*. In this famous guide, garlic is rated as being very high in starch. However, I have never found this to be true when testing with iodine. I use fresh garlic in cooking, inserting slivers into steaks and roasts, and simmer whole cloves in oil when making sauces. But I discard them before eating. Nevertheless, I use garlic granules (sometimes called garlic powder) frequently and find it an excellent way of adding flavour, for example sprinkled over roast chicken. It never causes me any problems. Do not confuse this with garlic salt. Garlic granules and garlic salt look very alike and often the packaging is so similar that it's easy to mistake one for the other. But garlic salt is *so* salty that you'll soon know the difference if you add it by mistake – the food will be inedible. You can now get crushed or puréed garlic in vegetable oil. I have tested this and it seems fine.

Dried herbs Experiment with the various types of mixed herbs now available, such as Italian, Mediterranean, Provençal, etc. They are often freeze-dried and have a very good flavour.

Fresh herbs The greatest flavour enhancer, and you can use them in so many dishes. Buy them planted in pots if you can as they stay fresh longer.

Lemons A drop or two of lemon juice is wonderful for bringing out the flavour of foods. A good trick is to pierce the lemon with a fine skewer or thick darning needle and just squeeze out the juice when you need it. This way it stays fresh far longer.

Olives I use canned or bottled, chopped or whole pitted black olives in sauces or casseroles. Both the olives and the liquor add a wonderful flavour dimension to certain dishes. A teaspoon of olive paste can also add zip to a dull sauce.

Fruit jellies   Try jelly jams such as redcurrant, blackberry, quince and strawberry. The best brand is Wilkin & Sons, Tiptree – not always readily available, but look for it in good supermarkets and speciality stores. All of these flavours are wonderful with hot or cold meats (yes, even the strawberry!) Mix them with mustard for a very good substitute for chutney.

Honey   Can be used in so many ways, in both sweet and savoury dishes. A dash adds flavour and colour to gravy. Runny honey in squeeze packs is more convenient.

Fruit sugar (proper name 'fructose')   Sometimes available in supermarkets and health food shops. Fruit sugar is slightly sweeter than ordinary sugar, and is a monosaccharide, so is easier to digest. It is very good in cooked fruit as it intensifies the fruity flavour. Some of my recipes may include fructose, but because it is not always available I have included the alternative of ordinary sugar as well. Use whichever you wish.

Ground almonds   This is the best starch-free substitute for flour that I have found. It is not really like flour in any way, except that it can look and taste quite similar. Ground almond makes good cakes and biscuits, although you won't be able to use it for light sponges, breads or sauces.

Fresh tomato stock cubes   See index for my own recipe for a mild, fruity, almost uncooked tomato sauce which I make in bulk and freeze in ice trays. When frozen, empty the cubes into plastic bags and store in the freezer.

Mustards   I use mustard more than any other condiment, in sauces and gravies. It can replace flavours and spices that I cannot eat. As long as you check the back of the jar for the addition of wheat flour (usually only in English mustards), it will be safe to use. I particularly like Dijon, but all the French and German mustards are excellent.

Mustard is produced from the seeds of three different types of plants, giving white (or yellow) mustard, black mustard and brown mustard. The most commonly known in this country are either English mustards made from white seeds and sold as dry powder or a paste, and French and German mustards, which are usually in paste form, mixed with wine or vinegar. American mustards, generally very mild, are also popular.

English mustards usually contain wheat flour, whether powder or paste, and I avoid these. The smooth type of French (Dijon), German or American mustards, however, do not contain any starch additives, although you should check the list of ingredients. You may see included in the list: 'mustard flour'. This is in fact ground mustard seed and not wheat flour, and is therefore safe to eat. Some Dijon and German mustards contain whole mustard seed, and some contain peppercorns. Beware of the latter.

All types of mustard can be used to flavour food, ranging from the sweet honey mustards to the salty, savoury flavour of Greek mustard with black olives. This can add a deeper taste to meat dishes – a bit like Marmite. It must be used with caution as it has a strong flavour. The honey mustard I often include in recipes is usually Honeycup, a Canadian brand, which is very mild and sweet. Just a little bit is an excellent addition to savoury sauces and gravies, because it helps replace the sweetish/savoury flavour of vegetables. You can make your own substitute by mixing a good Dijon mustard with honey, to taste.

Soups

Soups are among the most difficult dishes to include on a starch-free diet. Most soups contain starch whether they're made from meat and vegetable stocks or cream sauces. The range is therefore very limited for those of us with starch intolerance.

You will see I have included several made with tomatoes. I feel I should add a warning note at this point: I can't make up my mind about tomatoes – not the taste, which I love, but whether they contain enough starch to worry about.

Tomatoes are properly classified as a fruit and therefore should not contain starch. I've tested them in a number of ways – lightly grilled, lightly fried, cooked for an hour or so, cooked with liquid and without. Sometimes they show evidence of starch, sometimes not. Surprisingly, the less ripe they are, the less starch is in evidence – which is the opposite of bananas!

I was very confused about tomatoes for a long time, but according to *The Composition of Foods* (McCance and Widdowson, see page 256), tomato juice, tomatoes raw and grilled contain only a trace of starch, fried (in corn oil) they contain 0.1, canned they contain 0.2 and puréed they contain 0.3. This indicates to me that the more they are cooked, the more starch they develop. Obviously, therefore, if you use tomato purée or canned tomatoes in a recipe, you are already beginning from a higher starch basis and the longer you cook the tomatoes, the more starchy they may become. I would recommend, therefore, that fresh tomatoes or tomato juice be used, although a very small amount of tomato ketchup has never caused me any trouble.

I leave it to you to decide. If you begin to experience IBS symptoms after eating dishes with a large cooked tomato content, give them up. Any symptoms you may experience will not be dramatically bad, and this will all depend on how intolerant you are to starch. Raw tomatoes are, of course, completely safe.

Chicken and apple soup (lactose-free)

Ingredients   **Serves four**

   2 chicken breasts with bones and skin
   3 teaspoons chopped fresh rosemary
   3 teaspoons clear honey
   4 tablespoons olive oil
   3 teaspoons garlic granules
   juice half a lemon
   1 litre (approx. 2 pints) water
   1 teaspoon honey-mustard
   ½ teaspoon olive mustard (optional)
   1 teaspoon starch-free steak seasoning (optional)
   2 sweet apples
   1 tablespoon chopped parsley

Method

Mix together the rosemary, honey, oil, lemon juice and 2 teaspoons of the garlic granules and marinate the chicken breasts in this mixture overnight.

Simmer the marinated chicken breasts in the water for several hours until so tender that the meat is falling off the bones. Remove the chicken, extract the bones and discard.

Dice the meat and return it to the stock. Peel and grate the apples and add to the stock. Add the remaining teaspoon of garlic granules, mustards and steak seasoning. Bring to the boil and simmer for 30 minutes. Check the flavour – more honey-mustard may be added if desired – and serve with chopped parsley.

Tomato and salmon soup

Ingredients   **Serves five**

1 litre (approx. 2 pints) tomato juice
50 g (2 oz) butter
½ teaspoon garlic granules
pinch onion powder
3 teaspoons sugar
1 teaspoon lemon juice
105 g (4 oz) can pink salmon with juice
   cream and chopped parsley to garnish

Method

Process the tomato juice, salmon, garlic and onion powder in food blender until almost smooth but not quite. Pour into a saucepan over a low heat. Add the sugar, salt, butter and lemon juice. Stir gently until hot, adjusting seasonings to taste.

Serve with a swirl of cream and a sprinkle of chopped parsley.

Sotos' lemon fish soup/stew

To turn this into a really filling meal, add a grilled round of goat's cheese or Haloumi cheese to each bowl.

Ingredients   **Serves four**

425 ml (¾ pint) water
425 ml (¾ pint) apple juice
100 ml (4 fl oz) homemade chicken stock (see Handy hints, page 250)
1 tablespoon dried onion granules
2 teaspoons garlic granules
1 teaspoon honey-mustard
juice of 1 lemon
bunch coriander, oregano or parsley
salt
4 good-sized portions of cod or haddock steaks, frozen or fresh
more lemon juice to taste
2–3 tablespoons chopped parsley
Parmesan cheese

Method

Frozen fish should be defrosted before use. Chop the herbs, then combine all except the last four ingredients and bring to boil. Simmer for about an hour.

Wash the fish, remove any bones and add to the stock. Simmer for about 10–15 minutes or until the fish is cooked. Check the flavour, add more salt or lemon juice to taste.

Remove the fish, place it in a large serving dish, pour the soup over, then sprinkle with chopped parsley and Parmesan cheese.

Chilled cucumber and yoghurt soup

Ingredients   **Serves four**

550 g (1¼ lb) or 2 medium cucumbers, peeled, seeded and chopped
1 medium size ripe pear, chopped
220 g (8 oz) carton low-fat plain yoghurt
325 ml (12 fl oz) water
100 ml (4 fl oz) homemade chicken stock (see Handy hints, page 250)
4 tablespoons fresh basil leaves

Method

Blend or process all the ingredients until smooth. Cover and refrigerate for several hours before serving. This soup can be made up to two days ahead – store covered in the refrigerator.

Bouillabaisse

A genuine Mediterranean recipe which I have adapted – a meal in itself.

Ingredients   **Serves four to five**

100 ml (4 fl oz) olive oil
4 tablespoons dried onion granules
2 teaspoons garlic granules
500 g (1 lb) ripe tomatoes, peeled and chopped
½ teaspoon dried thyme or sprig fresh thyme
2 bay leaves
2 tablespoons orange juice
100 ml (4 fl oz) white wine
1 litre (approx. 2 pints) boiling water
salt
1 teaspoon honey-mustard or 1 teaspoon Dijon mustard and a
     dash of honey
1.5 kg (3 lb) fish

Method

Choose a selection of fish: conger or moray eel, gurnard, small monkfish tail, red mullet, small bream, small bass, John Dory – or if possible, Mediterranean varieties such as the spiny scorpion fish called rascasse and other small rockfish, spiny lobster, raw king prawns, scallops or calamari (ask your fishmonger to prepare any unfamiliar fish). Make sure the prawns are deveined but leave tails intact. Clean, cut and scale any unprepared fish.

Heat half the olive oil in large pan. Sauté the onion granules, garlic granules and bay leaves for a few seconds – don't allow to brown – then add the tomatoes and cook for 5 minutes.

Add the orange juice and thyme. Pour in the boiling water, increase the heat and stir well. Add the salt and the rest of the oil, boiling vigorously so that the oil is properly mixed. Add the wine, reduce the heat, taste and add more honey-mustard if too tart.

Add the fish in order of cooking time – check with your fishmonger which will take the longest – and simmer for 5–8 minutes. Lift each fish out as it becomes cooked and place in a heated serving dish (leave some softer fish to disintegrate into the broth). Pour broth over fish and serve, or eat as two separate courses.

Creamy tomato and bacon soup

Ingredients   **Serves four**

500 g (1 lb) fresh tomatoes or 450 ml (16 fl oz) tomato juice
125 g (4 oz) diced bacon
100 ml (4 fl oz) water
1 teaspoon honey-mustard (optional)
1–2 teaspoons sugar
½ teaspoon garlic granules
3 rounded tablespoons plain Greek yoghurt – either full or low-fat
chopped chives

Method
Gently cook the bacon in a soup pot. When tender, add the tomatoes, water, honey-mustard, sugar and garlic granules. Bring slowly to the boil and simmer, adjusting seasonings. Stir in the yoghurt, bring to the boil again and serve, sprinkled with chopped chives.

Gazpacho (lactose-free)

I have always loved this soup, but recently I discovered that the genuine Mediterranean recipe contains a slice or so of white bread, blended into the ingredients. This recipe, therefore, is an adaptation, and sadly I recommend that you ask the cook, before you eat the genuine article.

Ingredients   Serves three to four
2 small green peppers, deseeded
1 kg (2 lb) ripe tomatoes, peeled and deseeded
2 small or 1 large cucumber, peeled
2 garlic cloves, crushed
100 ml (4 fl oz) or less (to taste) best virgin olive oil
about 6 tablespoons (or less) wine vinegar (to taste)
salt
1 teaspoon sugar

Method
Place the tomatoes in a bowl and pour boiling water over them, wait a few minutes then skewer each one with a fork and peel. Cut into chunks and remove the seeds.

Put all the vegetables through a blender with the garlic. Add the olive oil, vinegar, salt and sugar. Blend to a light creamy consistency, adding a few tablespoons of iced water if necessary. Serve very cold accompanied by garnishes.

Garnishes
Dice 1 cucumber, 1 onion, 1 red pepper, 1 green pepper, 1 tomato and 2 boiled eggs finely and place in individual bowls so that a little of each can be sprinkled on the soup, as desired.

Cream of asparagus soup

Ingredients   **Serves four**

1 kg (2 lb) fresh asparagus
1.5 litres (2½ pints) water
100 ml (4 fl oz) homemade chicken stock jelly (see Handy hints, page 250)
1 egg yolk
125 ml (5 fl oz) crème fraîche
salt to taste

Method

Add the chicken stock to the water and blend well. Break the asparagus into small pieces and cook them in the stock for 30 minutes.

Remove from the heat when they are all soft and purée in a blender or rub through a sieve. Combine the egg yolk and crème fraîche, whisk into the purée, replace over a very low heat just to heat through, adjust seasonings and serve. May also be served cold.

Starters

Any of the dishes in this section can be served as starters or party food, either together or individually. Serve the pâtés and dips with raw vegetables for IBS people.

Asparagus gratin

Ingredients   **Serves two**
>   *500 g (1 lb) fresh asparagus*
>   *125 g (4 oz) butter*
>   *4–6 tablespoons grated Parmesan cheese*
>   *1 teaspoon salt*

Method

Snap off the tough stems of the asparagus. Place in a single layer in a large pot or pan with a small amount of water – not enough to cover the asparagus. Add salt. Simmer until just beginning to cook and still bright green – about 8–15 minutes, depending on thickness. Remove and allow to drain. Place in a gratin dish, melt the butter and pour over the asparagus, sprinkle over the grated cheese and brown under a preheated grill.

Tapenade (lactose-free)

Ingredients   **Makes one bowl**
>   *1 cup pitted black Spanish olives (in brine)*
>   *¼ cup capers*
>   *6 anchovy fillets*
>   *⅓ cup canned tuna*
>   *2 cloves garlic*
>   *pinch ground bay leaves*
>   *pinch dried thyme*
>   *1 teaspoon mild Dijon mustard*
>   *1 teaspoon cognac*
>   *1 teaspoon lemon juice*
>   *4 tablespoons chopped parsley*

Method

Drain the olives, capers, anchovy fillets and tuna. Peel the garlic. Put everything except the final three ingredients into an electric blender or food processor and purée. Stir in the cognac, lemon juice and parsley, season with black pepper to taste.

Gorgonzola mousse

Ingredients   Serves six

6 *eggs*
325 *ml (12 fl oz) whipping cream*
1½ *tablespoons (1½ sachets) gelatine*
4 *tablespoons cold water*
375 *g (13 oz) Gorgonzola cheese, blended or sieved until soft*
100 *ml (4 fl oz) double cream*
light cooking oil

Method

This looks very good made in an oblong dish. Prepare a dish to use as a mould, which should be at least 7.5 cm (3 inches) deep, and either 20.5 cm (8 inches) in circumference (round dish) or approximately 32.5 x 18.5 cm (12¾ x 7½ inches) for an oblong dish. Pour in a small amount of cooking oil and tilting the dish so that the oil spreads over the base and around the sides. Set aside. Sieve or blend the cheese until smooth.

Separate the eggs, placing all the yolks in a saucepan or the top of a double boiler. Reserve 3 of the whites in a separate bowl. Put 6 tablespoons of the whipping cream into the saucepan with the egg yolks. Whisk the egg yolks and cream over simmering water until thick, then remove from the heat. Pour the gelatine into a small bowl, add the four tablespoons of cold water and stir over simmering water until the gelatine is dissolved. Remove from the heat. Pour the gelatine mixture into the egg and cream mixture and stir well. Add the sieved cheese to the egg/cream/gelatine mixture and leave to cool.

Meanwhile, beat the egg whites until stiff and set aside. In a separate bowl, beat the remaining whipping cream and the double cream together until stiff and set aside. Fold the beaten egg whites and the cheese mixture into the whipped cream mixture. Pour all into the prepared dish, making sure beforehand that the oil still coats the sides. Chill in the refrigerator for at least 2 hours.

To unmould, upturn the dish on to a serving plate, wrap a teatowel that has been dipped in hot water and wrung out around the dish and wait for the mousse to slide out. Decorate with thinly sliced cucumber arranged over the top.

Crudités with aïoli sauce (lactose-free)

Ingredients   **Makes one bowl**
  2 egg yolks
  225 ml (8 fl oz) olive oil
  1 tablespoon lemon juice
  salt
  5 large cloves garlic
  selection of raw vegetable pieces – celery, tomatoes, cucumber, radishes, red
    and yellow peppers, carrot sticks, fennel, cauliflower and apple slices

Method
Slice both ends off each garlic clove and place on a chopping board. Squash with the blade of a heavy knife and skin will peel off easily. Purée the garlic in a blender or mortar with salt to taste and a little of the oil. Stir in the lemon juice.

In a separate bowl, beat the egg yolks until pale but not foamy, then add the remainder of the oil slowly, beating vigorously. Add garlic purée and more salt if desired.

Stand aside to allow flavour to mature. This is best made early in the day to serve in the evening.

Antipasto

When buying processed meats such as salami and garlic sausage, it is always best to buy pre-packed meats with a list of ingredients on the pack. Sadly, those made in the UK often have modified starch or other starches such as potato flour added. Most European-made varieties are starch-free.

On a large flat serving dish, arrange a selection of cold meats: salamis, various hams, garlic sausage, sliced smoked turkey breast, etc. Alternate with cheese cut into sticks or cubes, olives, strips of cucumber, red and green peppers, spring onions, anchovy fillets, prawns, tiny lettuce leaves and melon slices.

Marinated mushrooms (lactose-free)

Ingredients   **Makes one bowl**
  250 g (9 oz) button mushrooms
  100 ml (4 fl oz) olive oil
  3 tablespoons lemon juice
  ½ teaspoon garlic granules
  ¼ teaspoon salt
  2 tablespoons chopped parsley

Method

Wash the mushrooms and allow them to dry while preparing the marinade. Combine the oil, lemon juice, garlic granules and salt in a screw-top jar and shake well. Pour into a serving dish and add the chopped parsley. Remove the stalks from the mushrooms and slice thinly. Toss lightly in the marinade and allow to stand at least 4 hours or overnight.

To serve, remove the mushrooms from the marinade with a slotted spoon and place in a small serving dish. Delicious as an addition to a green salad.

Fromage blanc and anchovy dip

Ingredients   **Makes one bowl**

    500 g (1 lb) fromage blanc
    8 anchovy fillets
    2 level tablespoons capers
    1 teaspoon mild French mustard
    2 tablespoons chopped chives
    1 tablespoon chopped parsley

Method

Thoroughly beat the fromage blanc until it is smooth. Drain the anchovies (if they are packed in brine you should also rinse them), remove as much of the backbone as possible, chop and add to the fromage blanc with all the other ingredients, reserving a few of the chopped chives.

Refrigerate for a few hours and serve in a small dish, sprinkled with the remaining chives.

Onion dip

Ingredients   **Makes one bowl**

    1 small can Nestlé cream
    1 teaspoon vinegar
    1 teaspoon onion granules
    ¼ teaspoon salt

Method

Empty contents of the can into a small dish, add onion granules and salt, then mix well. A dash of tomato ketchup or a teaspoon of mild mustard can also be added, if desired.

Prosciutto and papaw (lactose-free)

Looks and tastes exotic and tropical – actually it is very easy and quick to prepare. Could also be used as a salad.

Ingredients   **Serves four**
 1 papaw
 ½ red pepper
 ½ green pepper
 4 tablespoons olive oil
 2 tablespoons dry white wine
 ½ clove garlic or ½ teaspoon garlic granules
 salt
 4 slices prosciutto ham – most supermarket deli sections stock this thin,
   darkish Italian raw dried ham nowadays, but if you can't get it,
   substitute thin slices of any ham.

Method
Cut the papaw into quarters and remove the seeds. Place on a serving dish and arrange a slice of ham over each quarter. Blend the oil, white wine, salt and crushed garlic well, or put all in a screw-top jar and shake. (Use your favourite vinaigrette dressing if you wish – just make sure it contains no modified starch.)

Slice the peppers thinly, place in a separate bowl, pour the dressing over and mix well. Place a spoonful of dressed peppers on top of the ham on each papaw slice and refrigerate until ready to serve.

Salmon pâté

Ingredients   **Makes one bowl**
 220 g (8 oz) can red salmon
 125 g (4 oz) pack cream cheese
 2 tablespoons lime or lemon juice
 1 tablespoon chopped chives
 100 ml (4 fl oz) any starch-free mayonnaise
 125 g (4 oz) melted unsalted butter

Method
Beat the cream cheese until soft. Add the drained salmon, chopped chives, mayonnaise and juice, and blend well. Add the melted butter, then blend until smooth. Spoon into a serving dish and refrigerate until set.

Cucumber and chive mousse

Ingredients   **Serves four**

   1 medium cucumber
   150 g (5 oz) cottage cheese
   85 ml (3 fl oz) Hellman's real mayonnaise (without modified starch)
   1 tablespoon finely chopped chives
   85 ml (3 fl oz) whipping cream
   ½ tablespoon (½ sachet) powdered gelatine
   4 tablespoons water
   1 rounded teaspoon caster sugar
   chopped parsley

Method
Beat the cottage cheese with an electric beater or blend until smooth.
Stir in the mayonnaise. Peel and quarter the cucumber lengthways,
remove the seeds and chop finely. Chop the chives. Add these to the
cottage cheese mixture.

   Put the water into a small saucepan, stir in the sugar. Sprinkle
the gelatine over the top, stir and allow to stand for a few moments.
Put the pan on a low heat and stir to dissolve. Remove and cool.

   Stir the cottage cheese mixture into the gelatine. Beat the cream
until stiff and fold into gelatine mixture. Spoon into small individual
ramekin dishes which have been lightly rubbed round with paper
towel dipped in cooking oil, and chill in the refrigerator until set.

   To serve, run a knife around inside of the ramekin to loosen the
mousse, upturn on to lettuce leaves and garnish with chopped
parsley.

Tuna mousse (lactose-free)

Ingredients   **Serves four**

   185 g (6 oz) can tuna in brine, drained
   2 tablespoons starch-free mayonnaise
   2 tablespoons lemon juice
   1 small onion finely chopped
   1 tablespoon chopped parsley
   1 tablespoon tomato purée
   ½ teaspoon French Dijon mustard
   ½ teaspoon honey-mustard
   3 teaspoons gelatine
   2 tablespoons water

Method

Blend the first eight ingredients until smooth. Put the water in a small saucepan and sprinkle the gelatine over. Allow it to stand for a few minutes and then gently dissolve, stirring well, over a low heat or over a pan of simmering water. Stir into the tuna mixture.

Rinse four individual ramekins or one larger serving dish with cold water – do not allow to dry. Spoon the mixture into the dish(es) and refrigerate for several hours or overnight. To serve, run a knife around the inside of the ramekins to loosen mousse and upturn, or upturn the larger dish wrapped in a tea towel dipped in hot water, until mousse slides out.

Veal and ham terrine (lactose-free)

So many bought pâtés and terrines contain breadcrumbs or modified starch. This recipe is a wonderful starter but also an ideal lunch dish with a salad.

Ingredients   **Serves six to eight as a starter**

 500 g (1 lb) veal steak
 275 g (10 oz) ham
 500 g (1 lb) ham fat
 275 g (10 oz) chicken livers
 1 tablespoon brandy
 3 bay leaves
 1 teaspoon dried onion granules
 1 teaspoon dried garlic granules
 25 g (1 oz) salted butter
 2 eggs
 2 teaspoons dried herbes de Provence or mixed herbs
 salt

Method

Marinate the chicken livers in the brandy for 30 minutes. Mince the veal, the ham and a quarter of the ham fat in a food processor or mincer in batches, until quite fine. Process the chicken livers with brandy until fine, or if using a mincer, drain, reserving brandy, and mince until fine. Add the livers and brandy to veal mixture.

Beat the eggs lightly and add to the meat mixture with the herbs, salt to taste. Melt the butter, stir in the onion and garlic granules, remove from the heat, add to the meat mixture and blend well.

Arrange the bay leaves in the base of a narrow, oven-proof dish or loaf tin (20 x 10 cm or 8 x 4 inches). Slice the remaining ham fat thinly and completely line the tin, allowing enough fat to overlap so that it can be folded over to cover the top. Pile the meat mixture into the tin and press down firmly, covering the top with overlapping fat. Cover with foil and place the whole container in a bain-marie (baking dish with hot water halfway up its sides) and bake in a moderate oven (180°C/350°F or gas mark 4) for 1½ hours.

Remove from the water, cool slightly and place a chopping board on top of the terrine, weighing it down with something heavy. When cold, refrigerate until required. Delicious served cold with bitter orange sauce (see index).

Simple scallops

Two easy recipes suitable as a starter for three, or main course for two.

Version one ingredients
12 scallops
50 g (2 oz) unsalted butter
garlic granules

Method
Sprinkle the scallops lightly with the garlic granules. Melt the butter in a heavy frying pan and when it begins to foam, add the scallops and cook for about 3–4 minutes each side. Serve with the hot garlicky pan juices poured over.

A richer sauce can be made (after removing the scallops to a warm plate) by blending a dash of dry white wine with the pan drippings and adding a tablespoon or so of double cream. Stir well and when it begins to bubble, pour over scallops.

Version two ingredients
12 scallops
juice 1 lime
4 tablespoons chopped fresh coriander leaves
50–75 g (2–3 oz) unsalted butter

Method
Melt the butter in a frying pan over a low heat, add the lime juice and coriander leaves and blend well. Turn up the heat and add the scallops. Cook for 3–4 minutes on each side, then serve with the pan juices poured over.

Show-off scallops

Ingredients   **Serves two to three**

12 or so scallops – depending on their size
garlic granules
50 g (2 oz) unsalted butter
100 ml (4 fl oz) brandy – apple or apricot brandy is good
150 ml (¼ pint) double cream
1 tablespoon chopped chives

Method

Sprinkle the scallops with the garlic granules. Melt the butter in a frying pan or chafing dish, add the scallops and cook over a high heat for 3 minutes on one side. Meanwhile, heat the brandy in a small saucepan. Remove the scallops from the heat, pour the brandy over the scallops, light the brandy with a match and, when it burns out, return the pan to a high heat and cook for 2 minutes. Add the cream, stir until hot again. Pour into serving dishes, then sprinkle with chopped chives.

Easy chicken liver pâté

Ingredients   **Serves four**

500 g (1 lb) chicken livers
85 ml (3 fl oz) brandy
90 g (3½ oz) butter
1 teaspoon onion granules
1 teaspoon garlic granules
85 ml (3 fl oz) double cream
salt
½ teaspoon dried mixed herbs

Method

Trim the livers and cut in half. Marinate in the brandy for at least 2 hours. Strain, reserving the liquid.

Melt half the butter in a pan, add the livers and cook for 3 minutes over a moderate heat. Add the brandy liquid and cook for a further minute. Remove from the heat, purée the liver in a blender or food processor. Melt the remaining butter, add the onion, garlic granules and mixed herbs, then add to the liver mixture and mix thoroughly. Add the cream and seasoning to taste. Place in a serving dish and refrigerate overnight.

Caviar pie

Ingredients   **Serves eight to ten as an entrée**
  8 large hard-boiled eggs
  75 g (3 oz) unsalted butter, melted
  170 ml (6 fl oz) thick soured cream
  100 ml (4 fl oz) Hellman's real or any starch-free mayonnaise
  1 teaspoon onion granules
  1 teaspoon sharp Dijon mustard
  100 ml (4 oz) jar caviar

Method
Finely chop the eggs and combine with the melted butter, mayonnaise, onion granules, mustard and 70 ml (2 fl oz) of the soured cream. Spread the mixture on to a quiche or pie plate. Spread the remaining 100 ml (4 fl oz) of soured cream over the top and chill overnight.

Before serving, spread the caviar evenly over the soured cream. Cut into slices and serve on lettuce leaves with lemon wedges.

Fresh goat's cheese with herbs

Ingredients   **Serves two to three**
  500 g (1 lb) fresh goat's cheese
  2 small spring onions
  1 wine glass full of dry white wine
  3 tablespoons olive oil
  2–3 tablespoons any or all of these herbs, finely chopped – parsley,
    chives, basil, chervil, tarragon, coriander

Method
Remove and discard the cheese skin or rind. Ideally, the cheese should be quite soft, but if it is more mature with a pungent aroma, add a little milk or single cream, blending it in with a fork until the texture is that of a fresh cheese. Add the olive oil and wine, then the finely chopped onions and herbs. Put in an airtight container and refrigerate for a few hours before serving. This recipe can be made a couple of days before use.

Smoked salmon curls

Ingredients   **Serves two to three**

   225 g (8 oz) smoked salmon
   4 tablespoons double cream
   225 g (8 oz) soft cream cheese with herbs
   50 g (2 oz) unsalted butter, softened
   1 tablespoon chopped chives

Method

Separate the thin slices of smoked salmon and spread them out on a layer of foil. Combine the remaining ingredients into a spreadable consistency and spread over the salmon. Roll up the salmon like a Swiss roll and wrap in the foil. Chill for 2 hours. Unroll and, with a sharp knife, slice and serve.

Tomato and mozzarella salad

Ingredients   **Serves six**

   5 beef tomatoes
   5 buffalo Mozzarella cheeses
   2 tins anchovy fillets
   fresh basil
   mild black Spanish olives in brine, pitted
   extra-virgin olive oil

Method

Slice the tomatoes and mozzarella thinly. Arrange on a large serving plate, overlapping the alternating tomato and cheese slices. Scatter the olives around the tomatoes, then drain the anchovy fillets and arrange on top.

   Tear off small basil leaves and arrange on top, or roughly chop larger basil leaves (they tend to discolour slightly when chopped). Drizzle with olive oil and serve.

Peppers with anchovy (lactose-free)

Ingredients   Serves six

2 orange peppers
2 red peppers
2 yellow peppers (or any other colour combination)
handful of fresh basil leaves
3 hard-boiled eggs
1 dessertspoon red wine or raspberry vinegar
3 tablespoons extra-virgin olive oil
100 g (4 oz) can of anchovy fillets
pitted or sliced black olives
rock salt

Method

Cut each pepper in half, remove the seeds and stalks. Put them skin side up under a very hot grill until black. Remove them, put them in a plastic bag and seal and lay aside. Remove yolks from eggs and sieve into a basin. Chop the egg whites finely. Take the peppers out of the plastic bag and peel the skins off. If they don't come off easily, leave them in the bag for a little longer. Lay the peppers out on a very large plate. Season with ground rock salt, sprinkle with the vinegar and pour the olive oil over. Sprinkle with the egg whites, followed by the basil and then the egg yolks. Chop the anchovy fillets in half and dot everything with the anchovies and olives. (Serve with crisp French bread for people who can eat starch.)

Chicken liver with basil pâté (lactose-free)

Ingredients   Serves eight to ten

500 g (1 lb) whole chicken livers
splash of cognac
1 teaspoon garlic granules or 2 cloves garlic, chopped
handful of fresh basil leaves
rock salt
175 g (6 oz) dairy-free spread such as Pure, or butter if you prefer (not
    lactose-free)

Method

Trim the livers of all the fatty or thready bits, place them in a single layer in an earthenware dish and sprinkle with cognac. It should not cover them, but they need to marinate in it for several hours. Turn from time to time so that both sides absorb the alcohol. Add the garlic and torn basil leaves and sprinkle with salt just before poaching. Gently poach the livers in their juice in a non-stick tin in the top of the oven, turning after a couple of minutes, until they are cooked on the outside but rosy pink within. Do not overcook. Tip into the blender with two-thirds (125 g/4 oz) of the dairy-free spread, and blend until smooth. Check the seasoning, then scrape into a terrine or loaf-size earthen-ware dish, and leave to cool. When cool, melt the remains of the spread, skim off any frothy scum, and pour over surface of pâté, placing a couple of fresh basil leaves in the centre. Put in the fridge until set. Remove from fridge a little while before serving with salad and/or hot toast.

Rare fillet steak with smoked oysters (lactose-free)

Ingredients   **Serves four to six**
   250 g (½ lb) or 2 medium-thick fillet steaks
   1 teaspoon olive oil
   2 x 65 g (2½ oz) cans smoked oysters
   salt
   diced fresh chives

Method
Heat a frying pan and add the oil. When it is almost smoking, add the beef fillets and fry for two minutes each side. Remove from heat and leave to cool. With a very sharp knife, slice the beef into thin slices. Season lightly with freshly ground rock salt. Place one or two smoked oysters on each slice, depending on the size of the oysters. Roll up the beef, secure with a cocktail stick if necessary. Place on serving plate and sprinkle with chives. Serve with a garnish of mixed dressed salad leaves.

Fish

Smoked haddock with cream

Ingredients   **Serves two**

   350 g (12 oz) smoked haddock
   250 ml (8 fl oz) double cream
   *freshly grated Parmesan cheese or, if preferred, 50–75 g (2–3 oz) of a mild
      cheese such as Emmental or Jarslburg*

Method

Bring just enough water to cover the fish to boil, then turn the heat
down. Add the fish and gently poach for about 5 minutes. Drain,
remove the skin, and flake the fish, removing any bones.

Butter an oven-proof dish, add the fish, pour over the cream and
sprinkle with grated cheese. Freshly grated Parmesan would be my
choice but you can use the packaged, pre-grated kind – or either of the
other cheeses mentioned above. Bake in a pre-heated oven at 200°C
(400°F or gas mark 6) for 20 minutes or until bubbling.

Mustard and honeyed fish

Ingredients   **Serves two**

   8 small fish fillets
   2 tablespoons grated Parmesan cheese
   2 teaspoons olive oil
   1 tablespoon lemon juice
   2 teaspoons French mustard
   1 teaspoon honey
   150 ml (¼ pint) water

Method

Make the sauce first. Combine the oil, lemon juice, mustard and honey
in a small saucepan. Stir in the water and simmer constantly over a low
heat, allowing the sauce to thicken.

Place the fish on a griller tray, sprinkle with half the cheese. Grill for
3 minutes and turn over, sprinkle with the remaining cheese, then grill
for a further 3 minutes. Serve with the sauce.

Salmon with dill (lactose-free)

Ingredients   **Serves two**

2 skinned, boned salmon fillets (more if small)
1 lemon
rock or sea salt
dairy-free spread, or butter (not lactose-free)
fresh dill

Method

Wash the dill and shake/spin dry. Prepare oven roasting dish by lining with foil. Squeeze lemon juice over foil, grind salt over the juice, dot with butter or spread. Lay salmon on foil. Repeat lemon juice, salt and butter/spread on top of the salmon. Lay the dill thickly over the top. Cover all with a sheet of roasting film cut from an oven roasting bag. Put in hot oven for about 15–20 minutes. Do not overcook. After 15 minutes, remove from oven, peel back roasting film and test by flaking with a fork. When still moist but just done, remove from oven. Remove all dill and place on serving dish. Spoon a little of the lemony juice over.

This dish can also be grilled. Proceed as above but sprinkle lightly with dried dill. Do not cover with roasting film. Place under hot grill until salmon is beginning to brown on top.

Fish with lime sauce

Ingredients   **Serves two**

4 medium-sized fish fillets of your choice – cod, coley, halibut, mullet are
    all suitable
85 ml (3 fl oz) fresh lime juice
4 tablespoons white wine vinegar
4 spring onions, chopped
1 teaspoon garlic granules
1 tablespoon sugar or honey
25 g (1 oz) butter, preferably unsalted
100 ml (4 fl oz) water
125 g (4 oz) extra butter

Method

Arrange the fish in a shallow dish in a single layer. Combine the lime juice, vinegar, sugar (honey), spring onions and garlic and pour over the fish. Cover and refrigerate for 2 hours. Remove the fish from the marinade, strain and reserve the liquid.

Heat 25 g (1 oz) butter in a frying pan, add the fish in a single layer and cook for about 4 minutes on each side or until cooked when tested with a fork. Remove the fish, place it in a serving dish and keep warm.

Heat the marinade in a small saucepan, add the water and bring to the boil. Reduce the heat and simmer uncovered until the mixture is reduced by about half. Chop the extra butter into small pieces and add slowly, whisking continuously until the sauce is thickish and smooth. Serve over the fish.

Danish fish with blue cheese

Ingredients   **Serves two**

2 slices fresh halibut
125 g (4 oz) butter
salt
50 g (2 oz) Danish blue cheese
1 tablespoon lemon juice
2 wedges lemon
chopped parsley

Method

Wash the fish and blot dry. Lightly sprinkle with salt and scatter several small pieces of butter on a flame-proof dish on which the fish is to be grilled and served.

Meanwhile melt the remaining butter, blue cheese and lemon juice together in a separate saucepan. Start to grill fish, basting with the cheese mixture. Continue cooking until the fish flakes when pricked with a fork or after about 7 minutes.

Serve sprinkled with parsley and decorated with lemon wedges.

Salmon with vermouth sauce

Ingredients   **Serves four**

4 medium salmon cutlets
675 ml (24 fl oz) water
75 ml (2½ fl oz) lemon juice
225 ml (8 fl oz) double cream
4 tablespoons dry vermouth
2 further teaspoons lemon juice
½ teaspoon garlic granules
1 tablespoon drained capers

1 *teaspoon chopped fresh thyme*
2 *tablespoons chopped fresh basil*
1 *teaspoon chopped fresh coriander*
1 *tablespoon chopped chives*

Method

Begin to make the sauce first. Chop all the fresh herbs ready to add to the sauce. Combine the cream and vermouth in a small saucepan and gently bring to the boil. Reduce the heat and simmer gently for about 10 minutes.

Meanwhile, combine the water and lemon juice in a large frying pan and bring to the boil, reduce the heat and poach the salmon for about 7 minutes or until just tender. Remove to a serving dish and keep hot. Add 2 further teaspoons lemon juice and the fresh herbs to sauce just before serving and stir to blend. Serve over cooked fish.

Smoked fish puff (lactose-free)

This dish is very low in calories.

Ingredients   Serves one

175 *g (6 oz) smoked haddock or other white smoked fish*
2 *teaspoons Heinz tomato sauce (or any starch-free ketchup)*
2 *medium eggs, separated*
dairy-free spread

Method

Flake the haddock, mix with the tomato sauce and egg yolks. Whisk the egg whites until stiff and fold into the fish mixture. Place in a small buttered oven-proof dish and cook for 15–20 minutes at a medium heat 180°C (350°F or gas mark 4). Serve with salad.

Smoked salmon omelette

This sounds expensive but it can be made quite cheaply from smoked salmon offcuts, often available from delis and supermarkets. Check to make sure they're a fresh, orangey-pink colour and moist, not hard and shiny.

Ingredients   **Serves one**
  50 g (2 oz) butter
  2 large eggs
  pinch salt
  4 tablespoons shredded smoked salmon trimmings
  1 tablespoon chopped parsley

Method
Whisk the eggs and salt with a fork until just blended. Melt half the butter in a small, heavy frying pan over a medium heat and put in the egg mixture. Reduce the heat and stir with a wooden spoon, making sure the eggs do not stick. Before the mixture cooks completely, take the pan off the heat, add the second piece of butter and smoked salmon, stir to blend and serve with chopped parsley.

Fish fillets with apricot sauce

Ingredients   **Serves six**
  6 large white fish fillets
  *425 g (15 oz) can or pack of apricot nectar or juice, or purée a can of
    apricot pieces*
  2 teaspoons onion granules
  2 teaspoons Greek yoghurt
  1 tablespoon fresh mint

Method
Place the fish in a lightly buttered baking dish. Combine the remaining ingredients and pour over the fish. Cover with a lid or foil. Bake in a moderate oven at 180°C (350°F or gas mark 4) for about 45 minutes or until the fish is tender.

Slimmer's seafood salad

Ingredients   **Serves two**

350 g (12 oz) white fish fillet
1 tablespoon lemon juice
½ teaspoon salt
1 large beefsteak tomato
125 g (4 oz) cucumber
2 tablespoons chopped chives
2 teaspoons capers
4–5 anchovy fillets
3 tablespoons natural low-fat yoghurt
1 tablespoon starch-free mayonnaise
1 teaspoon starch-free tomato ketchup
125 g (4 oz) peeled prawns
lettuce leaves for serving

Method

Wash and skin the fish and cut into cubes. Place in a single layer over the bottom of a wide saucepan or frying pan. Pour over enough water just to cover the fish. Add the lemon juice and salt and heat until the water is simmering. Poach gently for 10–15 minutes, or until cooked. Drain and allow to cool.

Dice the tomato and cucumber and mix with capers and chopped chives. Dice the anchovy fillets and mix with the mayonnaise, yoghurt and tomato ketchup. Toss the fish cubes into the salad vegetables. Line a serving plate with lettuce leaves. Pile the fish mixture on to the leaves, then pour the dressing over. Scatter prawns on top and serve.

Crusty fish fillets

Ingredients   **Serves four**

4 large white fish fillets
2 tablespoons lemon juice
1 tablespoon dry white wine
75 g (3 oz) ground (blanched) almonds
125 g (4 oz) grated mild cheese
2 teaspoons Dijon coarse-grain mustard
2 tablespoons chopped fresh parsley
1 tablespoon chopped fresh chives
1 tablespoon chopped fresh dill
1 teaspoon garlic granules
50 g (2 oz) melted butter

Method
Place the fish fillets in single layer in a lightly greased oven-proof dish, sprinkle with the lemon juice and wine. In a small bowl, combine the remaining ingredients and spoon evenly over the fish. Bake uncovered in a moderate oven at 180°C (350°F or gas mark 4) for about 40 minutes or until the fish is tender when tested with a fork.

Baked fish with herb butter pockets

Ingredients   Serves six
  6 small whole fish or portions of a large whole fish
  275 g (10 oz) salted butter
  4 bacon rashers
  4 tablespoons chopped fresh parsley
  1 tablespoon chopped fresh chives
  1 tablespoon chopped fresh thyme
  4 tablespoons Parmesan cheese
  1 teaspoon garlic granules
  ½ teaspoon onion granules
  1 tablespoon lemon juice

Method
The fish should be boned but left as whole as possible. Dice the bacon. Beat the butter in a small bowl until creamy, then add the bacon, herbs, cheese, garlic, onion and lemon juice. Blend well. Spread the mixture on the inside of the fish and wrap each serving in foil.

Bake in an oven-proof dish in a moderate oven at 180°C (350°F or gas mark 4) for about 30 minutes or so, depending on the size of the fish (peel back the foil and test with a fork for tenderness). Serve with lemon wedges. This can also be cooked on a barbecue.

Salmon pizza-ish

Ingredients   Serves two
  225 g or 8 oz can pink salmon
  2 tablespoons double cream
  several tomatoes – the sweeter the better, any size will do
  1–2 teaspoons garlic granules
  1–2 teaspoons dried mixed herbs or Italian herbs
  ½–1 cup grated mild Cheddar
  ½ dozen pitted black olives and/or strips of salami

Method

Drain the salmon and turn into a small gratin dish. Press it evenly over the bottom. Dribble double cream all over the salmon. Slice the tomatoes and arrange in a layer over the salmon. Sprinkle with the garlic granules. Grate the cheese and spread over the tomatoes. Sprinkle with dried herbs. Slice the olives and/or salami and arrange over the cheese. Cook in a hot oven at 220°C (425°F or gas mark 7) until it looks like a cooked pizza.

Creamy salmon bake

Ingredients   **Serves two**

 1 medium 225 g or 8 oz can and 1 small 125 g or 4 oz can pink salmon
 4 rashers bacon
 350 ml (12 fl oz) whipping cream
 3 eggs
 1 tablespoon grated Parmesan cheese
 2 tablespoons chopped parsley

Method

Dice the bacon and fry gently until crisp. Drain the salmon, reserving the liquid, flake, remove the bones and spread evenly on the bottom of a medium-sized oven-proof dish.

Beat the cream until thick. In a separate bowl beat the eggs until thick and creamy. Fold the cheese, salmon liquid and parsley into the egg mixture and blend well. Fold in the cream.

Sprinkle the diced bacon over the salmon. Pour the egg mixture over the top. Bake in a moderately hot oven at 190°C (375°F or gas mark 5) for 10 minutes. Reduce the heat to moderately low 170°C (325°F or gas mark 3) and bake for a further 30–35 minutes, or until the bake is set and beginning to brown on top.

Poultry and game

Lemon-garlic chicken strips in cream sauce

You can serve the chicken without the sauce if you're trying to cut down on calories.

Ingredients   **Serves two**

  4 boneless chicken breasts
  lemon juice
  2 teaspoons garlic granules
  25 g (1 oz) butter
  olive oil for frying
  2 tablespoons crème fraîche or Greek yoghurt
  ½ teaspoon sugar
  100 ml (4 fl oz) white wine or water
  salt to taste
  handful chopped parsley

Method
Remove any gristle or fat from the chicken breasts and slice each breast into 4 or 5 thinnish strips. Place on a plate and squeeze the lemon juice over, turning and making sure both sides are coated in juice. Sprinkle one side liberally with garlic granules.

Heat the olive oil and butter in a frying pan over a high heat. Drop the chicken, garlic-side down, into oil and butter and fry quickly for about 3 minutes. Just before turning sprinkle with the remaining garlic. Turn and fry for about 3–5 minutes depending on thickness (test with a fork to make sure the chicken is just cooked – do not overcook).

Remove from heat and place the chicken in a serving dish. Keep warm. Pour excess oil and butter from the pan and replace on a low heat. Add the sugar and wine, stir until dissolved and all the brownings from the pan are scraped off. Add salt to taste. Cook for a few minutes until mixture thickens slightly. Add crème fraîche or Greek yoghurt and stir well until the sauce reaches the desired thickness. More wine or water can be added if necessary.

Pour the sauce over the chicken strips. Add the parsley and serve.

Chicken Marsala

Ingredients   **Serves four**
> 4 large or 3 small skinless chicken breasts
> 25 g (1 oz) butter
> olive oil
> 1–2 teaspoons garlic granules
> 4 anchovy fillets
> 12 capers
> 4–8 slices mozzarella cheese
> 1 tablespoon chopped parsley
> 3 tablespoons Marsala wine
> 150 ml (¼ pint) cream
> salt

Method
Remove any gristle or fat from the chicken breasts and sprinkle with garlic granules. Melt the butter in a pan with enough olive oil for frying, then add the chicken breasts and cook for a few minutes on each side until lightly browned and almost cooked through. Remove the pan from the heat.

Lay a slice of cheese over each breast and top each with an anchovy fillet, three capers and a sprinkle of parsley. Return the pan to moderate heat and cook a further 5 minutes. Remove from the pan and place the chicken in a serving dish. Keep warm.

Add Marsala to the pan drippings and return to the heat. Scrape the pan brownings off the bottom, reduce the heat, add the cream and simmer gently for a few minutes until sauce thickens. Season to taste with salt.

Pour over the chicken breasts and serve.

Roast chicken with lemon and herb sauce

This simple way to roast chicken is my family's favourite. I've discovered that the large family-size bird is usually the most tender, so I often cut one in half, right down the centre, and then cook one half (which serves three) and freeze the other. The chicken must be roasted alone. Roast vegetables in a separate dish, using the herby chicken/butter fat from a previous roasting.

Ingredients   **Serves three to six**
  any size chicken
  ½ a lemon
  garlic granules
  75 g (3 oz) butter
  2 fresh bay leaves and 2 sprigs fresh rosemary or sprinkle of dried herbs

Sauce (optional)
  1–2 teaspoons honey-mustard
  slosh white wine or water
  2 tablespoons Greek yoghurt or crème fraîche
  salt

Method
Place the chicken in a roasting or oven-proof dish. Squeeze the half lemon over the chicken, then place the lemon in the cavity inside the chicken. Sprinkle the chicken with garlic granules. Press thin slices of butter all over the chicken breast and legs. Push the fresh herbs into the cavity so that they are just sticking out, or press them over the top of chicken (or sprinkle the chicken with dried herbs).

Cover with foil or a roasting bag and place in a moderate oven at 180°C (350°F or gas mark 4) for 1 to 1½ hours. Remove from oven and check for 'doneness' (if the juices run clear when prodded with a fork, it is cooked). If it is not cooked enough, return to the oven with the foil removed to allow browning.

When cooked, remove the chicken from oven, place it on an oven-proof dish and stand in warm place. Skim the fat from the roasting dish by standing it on a tilt and allowing the thick chicken stock to settle to the bottom. With a large, flat spoon, gently skim off the clear fat, reserving it in a clean jam jar. When you have skimmed off as much fat as you can, place the roasting dish with the remaining chicken stock on a very low heat. Stir in the honey-mustard, scraping any brownings from the edge of the pan. Add the wine or water and stir, tasting and adding salt as desired. Add the yoghurt and stir to blend, until the sauce begins to thicken. Serve the sauce as gravy.

If you don't want to make the sauce, reserve the remaining chicken stock in a jar or freeze in ice-cube containers.

Chicken kebabs

You need to soak the kebab skewers in water for about an hour before cooking, to prevent burning.

Ingredients   **Serves two or three**
   3 large skinless chicken breasts
   2 tablespoons no-starch vinaigrette or French dressing
   1 tablespoon orange juice
   1 tablespoon lemon juice
   1 tablespoon water
   2 tablespoons grated Parmesan cheese
   2 tablespoons chopped fresh basil
   2 tablespoons chopped fresh parsley
   2 tablespoons chopped chives

Method
Remove any gristle or fat from the chicken and chop into 2½ cm (1 inch) chunks. Combine all the other ingredients in a bowl, add chicken and marinate, refrigerated, for at least an hour. Remove the chicken, reserving the marinade. Thread the chicken on to skewers and grill on both sides under high heat, basting frequently with marinade, until cooked.

Orange-minty chicken

Ingredients   **Serves four**
   4 large skinless chicken breasts
   4 tablespoons chopped fresh mint
   100 ml (4 fl oz) white vinegar
   225 ml (8 fl oz) orange juice
   1 tablespoon sugar
   50 g (2 oz) butter

Method
Flatten the chicken breasts with a meat mallet or a rolling pin until thin. Scatter the mint evenly over each fillet and roll up tightly, securing with a cocktail stick. Bake covered in an oven-proof dish in moderate oven at 180°C (350°F or gas mark 4) for about 25 minutes or until the chicken is tender.

Meanwhile make the sauce. Combine the vinegar and sugar in a small saucepan, stirring over a low heat until the sugar is dissolved.

Bring it to the boil, then boil rapidly without stirring until the mixture turns a light golden brown. Add the orange juice and bring to the boil again. Reduce the heat and simmer until reduced by about half. Add butter and stir until blended.

Remove the cooked chicken from the oven, remove the cocktail sticks and slice into rounds. Serve with sauce.

Cheese stuffed chicken breasts

Ingredients   Serves four
4 large skinless chicken breasts
125 g (4 oz) cottage cheese
2 tablespoons chopped chives
1 teaspoon dried tarragon leaves
1 tablespoon (approximately) jellied chicken stock (see Handy hints, page
    250)
225 ml (8 fl oz) water

Sauce
100 ml (4 fl oz) water or stock
2 tablespoons lemon juice
2 teaspoons sugar
25 g (1 oz) butter
1 tablespoon plain yoghurt

Method
Remove any gristle or fat from the chicken breasts and cut a pocket in the thickest part. Press the cottage cheese through a sieve and combine with the chives and tarragon. Stuff pockets with this mixture. Place the breasts in an oven-proof dish. Combine the stock and water, pour over the chicken and bake, covered, for about 20 minutes in a moderate oven at 180°C (350°F or gas mark 4). Remove from the heat, place the chicken on a serving plate and keep warm.

Measure the remaining liquid and make it up to 100 ml (4 fl oz) with additional water if necessary. Add the lemon juice, sugar, butter and yoghurt. Blend over a medium heat just until it thickens. Serve over the chicken.

Cary's rich cream and brandy chicken casserole

Ingredients   **Serves three to four**

1 large pre-cooked chicken or 6 pre-cooked breasts (cold)
soft dried apricots
450 ml (16 fl oz) fresh orange juice and grated zest of 1 large orange
segments of 1 large orange
sprinkle of mixed Italian herbs
100 ml (4 fl oz) double cream
225 ml (8 fl oz) white wine
4 tablespoons brandy

Method

Pull whole chicken into serving size pieces or arrange breasts in ovenproof dish. Wash and zest the orange (grate outside of orange taking care only to get the orange zest, not any of the pale, bitter pith), then peel and divide the segments. Combine the orange juice, zest, apricots and orange segments. Pour all over chicken. Sprinkle with mixed herbs and cook, covered, in a moderate oven at 180°C (350°F or gas mark 4) for 20–30 minutes or until completely warmed through. Blend the cream with the wine. Remove the chicken from the heat and pour cream and wine over, blending with the juices and basting the chicken well. Turn up the heat and cook in hot oven at 200°C (400°F or gas mark 6) for further 10 minutes. Remove from the heat and add the brandy (a good slosh). Blend into the sauce and serve.

Slimmer's simple chicken (lactose-free)

So easy and delicious. I usually make twice as much as I need and slice or cube the cold chicken into a salad the next day.

Ingredients

chicken breasts – 1 or 2 for each person
1 lemon
garlic granules (optional)

Method

Remove any skin and gristle or fat from the chicken. Sprinkle lemon juice lightly over both sides of each breast. Place each breast on a piece of foil and sprinkle with garlic granules (if desired). Fold the foil around each breast and place in an ovenproof dish. Cook for 20–25 minutes in a hot oven at 190°C (375°F or gas mark 5). Don't overcook –

open one parcel and check for 'doneness' at 20 minutes. If you plan to use any of the chicken cold, leave it in the foil until the next day as it improves the flavour.

Breast of chicken in rum crumbs

Ingredients   **Serves two**

2 *large skinless chicken breasts*
4 *tablespoons ground almonds*
5 *tablespoons rum*
1 *tablespoon strawberry or blackberry or black cherry jelly (jam jelly)*
1 *teaspoon honey-mustard*
50 *g (2 oz) butter*
olive oil for frying

Method
Flatten each chicken breast with a rolling pin, meat mallet or the edge of a saucer until thin. Place the ground almonds on a plate. Pour 4 tablespoons of rum into a shallow dish, dip the chicken breasts in it and then dip them in the ground almonds.

Over a medium heat, melt the butter, add the olive oil and sauté each chicken slice for a few minutes each side, or until golden. Meanwhile, combine the jelly, honey-mustard and a tablespoon of rum over a low heat. Place the chicken on a serving dish, pour the sauce over and serve.

Roast chicken with mustard (lactose-free)

Ingredients   **Serves four**

4 *large chicken pieces including bone and skin*
4 *level tablespoons Dijon coarse-grain mustard*
4 *sprigs of fresh herbs – such as rosemary or sage or lemon balm*
8 *rashers of bacon*

Method
Arrange the chicken pieces in an oven-proof dish, spread mustard over each, add a sprig of fresh herbs and cover each with two rashers of bacon. Bake in a hot oven at 220°C (425°F or gas mark 7) for 25 minutes. May also be grilled or barbecued.

French roast chicken

Ingredients
Serves four to six

family-sized roasting chicken
approximately 90 g (3½ oz) salted butter
2 tablespoons chopped parsley
1 teaspoon chopped tarragon
1 teaspoon Dijon mustard
2 fresh bay leaves
2 sprigs fresh rosemary
225 ml (8 fl oz) water
100 ml (4 fl oz) white wine

Method
Beat the butter until soft. Add the parsley, tarragon and mustard and blend well. With your fingers, gently ease the skin away from chicken breast. Spread the butter mixture over the meat underneath the skin, covering as much of the breast as you can. Pull the skin back to cover the meat completely.

Put the chicken on a baking dish. Stuff the bay leaves and rosemary into the chicken cavity. Blend the water and wine, then pour it over the chicken and cook uncovered, basting frequently, in a moderate oven at 180°C (350°F or gas mark 4) for about 1½ hours or until the juices run clear when the chicken is pierced with a fork. Make a gravy from the pan juices (see index).

Chicken apple casserole

Ingredients
Serves four

1 large chicken
50 g (2 oz) butter
2 teaspoons garlic granules
2 sweet apples
2 teaspoons honey-mustard
300 ml (½ pint) apple juice
1 teaspoon vinegar
1 tablespoon plain mild yoghurt
salt
1 tablespoon double cream
handful chopped parsley

Method

Untruss the chicken and sprinkle with garlic granules. Melt the butter in a frying pan and brown the chicken gently on both sides. Remove the pan from the heat. Place the chicken in a deep casserole dish (preferably with a lid) which is not too much larger than the bird, so that the juices can nearly cover it while cooking.

Peel and slice the apples into thick chunks. Return the pan to the heat and fry the apple chunks gently in the pan brownings. Remove from the heat and add the apple chunks to the casserole dish with the chicken. Return the pan to a low heat.

Stir in the honey-mustard, apple juice, vinegar and yoghurt, blending well with the brownings from the pan. Add salt to taste. Pour over chicken, cover and cook 1–1½ hours in a moderate oven at 180°C (350°F or gas mark 4), basting several times. When done, the chicken juices will run clear when the meat is pierced.

Remove the chicken to a serving plate and keep warm. Pour the sauce, including the apple chunks, into a small pan over a low heat. With a potato masher, mash the apple chunks as finely as possible – you can do this in a blender, but I rather like the slightly chunky texture of the masher method. Increase the heat and boil until reduced. Add a tablespoon of double cream (more if you wish) and boil until thick. Check the seasonings. Throw in a handful of chopped parsley and serve over the chicken.

Elizabeth David's poached chicken

Ingredients   **Serves four to six**
   1 *medium to large chicken*
   50 g (2 oz) *butter*
   2 *egg yolks*
   225 ml (8 fl oz) *cream*
   bunch tarragon
   lemon
   salt

Method
Cut the lemon in half and rub the outside of the chicken with the juice. Chop the tarragon. Blend the butter with 1 tablespoon of the tarragon, add salt to taste and put inside the chicken. Place the chicken in a large saucepan and pour over enough water to barely cover it. Poach the chicken gently, uncovered, basting frequently with the liquid, until it is cooked. Leave it to cool in the stock. When cooled, remove the chicken to a deep serving dish.

Strain the stock. Beat the yolks of the eggs with the cream and another tablespoon of chopped tarragon. Heat about ½ pint of the stock in a small pan, pour a spoonful or two on to the egg and cream mixture, then pour it all back into the pan, stirring continuously until the sauce thickens, but do not make it too thick as it will continue to solidify as it cools.

Pour this over the chicken in the dish and leave it to get cold. Serve decorated with whole tarragon leaves.

Baked orange chicken

Ingredients   Serves four
4 *chicken portions, with skin, on the bone*
50 g *(2 oz) butter*
225 ml *(8 fl oz) orange juice*
1 *dessertspoon dried onion granules*
1 *tablespoon homemade chicken stock (see Handy hints, page 250)*
100 ml *(4 fl oz) water*
1 *teaspoon dried tarragon*
salt

Method
Melt the butter in a frying pan and brown the chicken lightly on both sides. Remove from the heat and place the chicken in a casserole dish. Return the pan to the heat, add chicken stock, orange juice, water, onion granules and tarragon. Stir to blend. Bring to the boil and remove immediately. Pour the sauce over the chicken, cover and cook in a moderate oven at 180°C (350°F or gas mark 4) for 1 hour or until the chicken is tender.

Tarragon-marinated chicken breasts (lactose-free)

The different vinegars give this dish a subtle deliciousness.

Ingredients   **Serves two to three**
  6 *chicken breasts, boned and skinless*
  4 *tablespoons extra-virgin olive oil*
  2–3 *tablespoons different vinegars (red wine, raspberry, sherry, white*
      wine, balsamic, etc., or you could use just one)
  1 *tablespoon smooth Dijon mustard*
  a large bunch fresh tarragon (about 75 g/3 oz) or 2 tablespoons dried
      tarragon

Method
Wash fresh tarragon, shake/spin dry. Place oil, vinegars and mustard into a mixing bowl and whisk together for a few minutes. Chop tarragon and add to oil mixture. There is no need to discard stems unless extremely woody – they have a good flavour. Add chicken and marinate for at least an hour, unrefrigerated. Can be marinated in fridge the day before or overnight. Cook at high heat on heavy cast-iron stove-top griddle, or on a barbecue. Can be cooked in heavy frying pan at high heat or directly on the bottom of the Aga roasting oven.

I sometimes make double the quantity of this and freeze half. For freezing, it is best to make a sauce to cover the chicken. You will need to cook the chicken in the frying pan and use additional ingredients to make the sauce:

  bottle good white wine
  any left-over marinade
  2 *knobs dairy-free spread, or butter (not lactose-free)*
  dash mild runny honey (optional)
  rock or sea salt

When cooked, remove the chicken to be frozen. Place in tinfoil container and set aside. Remove the rest of the chicken to a serving plate and keep warm. Add half or three-quarters of the wine to the pan, scraping any brownings from the edge of the pan. Simmer gently. Add marinade to the pan liquid and stir. Check for flavour, add salt and dash of honey if required. Allow to reduce until beginning to thicken slightly. Add knobs of spread/butter and stir. Pour over chicken in foil packs. Cool and freeze.

Roast chicken with vinegar (lactose-free)

Ingredients   **Serves two to three**

medium-size free-range corn-fed chicken
1 tablespoon mild vinegar (raspberry or red/white wine)
garlic granules
50 g (2 oz) dairy-free spread
about a tablespoon dried tarragon
2–3 teaspoons Dijon mustard
water
dash mild runny honey

Method
Remove chicken from packaging and place (trussed) in roasting dish. I prefer a roasting dish with a lid, but this is not necessary. Carefully drizzle the vinegar over the chicken legs and breast as best you can, to give a thin covering. Scoop up any dribbles that fall to the bottom of the pan and baste any parts that you have missed. Sprinkle all over with garlic salt. Place the dairy-free spread in a saucer and sprinkle thickly with dried tarragon. Blend together. With the flat of a knife, spread the tarragon mixture over the breast and legs of the chicken. Cover with a roasting bag sliced down one side and turned into a 'tent', and tuck in at the sides, or with lid.

Place in a hot oven 220°C (425°F, gas mark 7) for 45–50 minutes. Remove from oven and check for 'doneness' (if the juices run clear when prodded with a fork, it is cooked). If it is not cooked enough, return to the oven for about 5–10 minutes. Remove and place on warm serving dish and keep warm.

Tilt the roasting pan at an angle until the thick stock settles and skim all the fat off with a large flat spoon. (Don't put the fat down the drain – put it into an empty jam jar.) Add enough water to the pan to cover the pan drippings. Stir, scraping any brownings from the edge of the pan. Add the Dijon mustard and blend. Taste and add a dash of honey if desired. The tarragon gives this dish a wonderful flavour – you may not need any honey. Simmer until slightly thickened. Carve the chicken and serve with the gravy. Add roast vegetables for others. Delicious with a salad.

Chicken with mustard sauce (lactose-free)

Terribly easy. Can be frozen and reheated.

Ingredients   **Serves any number**
   any amount of chicken thighs or drumsticks including skin
   Dijon mustard
   wine or grape juice
   dash mild runny honey (optional)
   olive oil

Method
Brown the chicken on each side in a frying pan with a very small amount of olive oil (or without any if using a non-stick pan). Pour off excess fat. While still in the pan, roughly coat one side of the chicken pieces with Dijon mustard. Turn and coat the other side. Pour over the wine or grape juice to barely cover the chicken. Cook over low heat, partially covered – place a lid on the pan but lift it at one end so that steam escapes. During the cooking, turn the pieces and coat with a little more mustard. Reduce the wine/mustard sauce until thick – this may mean lifting the lid and cooking uncovered at times, but the sauce thickens very quickly when uncovered. Add more wine if it becomes too thick. When the chicken is tender, taste the sauce and add a dash of honey if desired. Serve.

Chicken with olives (lactose-free)

Another chicken recipe with similar ingredients, but all have a slightly different taste. You will learn to experiment with your own variations.

Ingredients   **Serves two**
   4 chicken breasts with skin
   about a dozen marinated olives (see Snacks, page 251)
   Dijon mustard
   3–4 rashers thin bacon, diced
   slosh of light vinegar (raspberry/red wine, etc.)
   dry or medium white wine
   1 teaspoon mild runny honey

Method
Fry diced bacon and remove. Fry chicken skin-side first, until fat runs off. Drain fat, turn and fry on skinless side. Paste skin-side with about a teaspoon of mustard for each breast. Turn and paste skinless side.

Add slosh of vinegar and then white wine to nearly cover, then add olives and bacon and stir, basting chicken. Add about a teaspoon of honey. Cover and simmer over low heat until sauce is thick. Add more honey to taste if desired.

Chicken with sage and Parma ham (lactose-free)

Ingredients   Serves two
4 large skinless chicken breasts
4 large slices Parma ham
bunch/packet fresh sage
about 18 marinated olives (see Handy hints, page 250)
dry white wine
about 1 teaspoon honey-mustard
3–4 fresh tomato stock cubes (see index)

Method
Depending on thickness of chicken breasts, either butterfly (slice down through thickest part and open out) or beat until flat with a meat mallet or (even better) the edge of a saucer. Lay slice of Parma ham over each. Dice olives and fresh sage, mix together. Spread a little of the mixture over each breast. Roll up and pin with cocktail sticks. Brown in olive oil on high heat. Remove to low heat, add wine, tomato stock cubes, honey mustard and remainder of olive/sage mixture. Cook covered either on top of cooker or in oven until tender.

Guinea fowl with prunes (lactose-free)

Guinea fowl are amazingly economical, as although they look quite small, they're very meaty and one bird can serve three to four people. Don't substitute chicken – its flavour is too delicate. Left-overs taste even better, reheated the next day, or can be frozen.

Ingredients   Serves six to eight
2 guinea fowl
dash vinegar
bottle red or white wine or red/white grape juice
225 g (8 oz) smoked streaky bacon, diced
225 g (8 oz) soft pitted prunes
Dijon mustard
honeycup mustard (optional)
olive oil

Method

Soak prunes in wine/grape juice for several hours or overnight. Cut each fowl into four. Dice bacon. Heat a little oil in a heavy stainless-steel or enamel casserole with lid. Brown bacon and remove. Brown fowl in batches. Return pieces of fowl to casserole in layers. Spread Dijon mustard roughly over each piece and sprinkle with bacon. Remove prunes with slotted spoon and layer over meat. Pour wine/grape juice over all, cover and put in hot oven 220°C (425°F, gas mark 7). Guinea fowl cooks quite quickly – check after about an hour. Remove from oven. Roughly stir ingredients. If desired, a couple of teaspoons of honeycup mustard can be added at this stage, to deepen the flavour and thicken the sauce. Serve.

Rabbit with prunes (lactose-free)

Ingredients   **Serves two to three**

   1 *rabbit*
   225 g (8 oz) *soft pitted prunes*
   1 *bottle red wine*
   2 *tablespoons olive oil*
   salt
   1 *tablespoon dried onion pieces*
   2 *teaspoons garlic granules*
   6 *rashers smoked streaky bacon*
   1 *bouquet garni – fresh if possible*

Method

Cover the prunes with the wine and soak for at least 2 hours beforehand. Cut the rabbit into serving size pieces, then brown them in the oil in a frying pan. Remove the pan from the heat and place the rabbit in a casserole dish.

Cut the bacon into small pieces, return the pan to the heat and brown the bacon in the oil. Add the dried onion and garlic to the pan and cook over a low heat for a few seconds only, then pour the wine from the prunes into the pan and stir to blend the pan browning with the liquid. Turn the heat up and leave to reduce (de-glaze) cooking juices until they thicken.

Pour the prunes over the rabbit, place the bouquet garni on top and pour the pan juices over all. Cover and cook in a moderate oven (180°C, 350°F, gas mark 4) for at least 2 hours. This dish can be cooked at a lower heat if necessary – just allow extra time. It is even better cooked the day before and reheated.

Turkey schnitzel (lactose-free)

Ingredients
1 turkey breast for each person
1 lemon
garlic granules
1 egg beaten with a little water
ground almonds
oil for cooking

Method
Place each turkey breast between clingfilm and flatten with a heavy object such as a rolling pin or the back of a heavy frying pan.

Beat the egg with the water in a wide-based dish. Pour the ground almonds on to a separate plate. Lay the turkey breasts on another plate and squeeze lemon juice over them. Turn and coat both sides. Sprinkle both sides with garlic granules. Dip each breast into the egg mixture and then into the ground almonds. Heat the oil in a heavy-based frying pan, and fry each schnitzel over a moderate heat until golden brown and completely cooked through. Serve with a slice of lemon.

Roast turkey with stuffing

Turkey is now available in so many sizes and prices, not to mention varieties, that it doesn't have to be kept for special occasions. This recipe is for a small, low-priced turkey, the sort you might have for a change for Sunday lunch or a dinner party. It cost me less than a joint of beef or leg of lamb. The long slow cooking is guaranteed to give you a moist, succulent result. The stuffing recipe is the same as I use at Christmas, but the amounts given are for a small turkey. Just double the ingredients for a large, Christmas-sized bird.

Ingredients   Serves four to six
fresh standard grade supermarket turkey about 3 kg (6½ lb)
    (the one I cooked was 6 lb 7½ oz or approximately 3.5 kg)
150 g (5 oz) stoned soft eating prunes
250 g (9 oz) soft dried apricots
300 g (11oz) (about 3 medium-sized) eating apples
3 tablespoons dried mixed herbs – any sort
1 teaspoon garlic Italian seasoning (optional)
¼ teaspoon onion salt
¼ teaspoon onion granules

1 teaspoon garlic granules
sprinkle of salt
2 eggs
about 1 tablespoon garlic granules extra
125–175 g (4–6 oz) butter
4 sprigs fresh rosemary and 4 fresh bay leaves (optional)

Method
Chop the dried fruit finely and place in a large mixing bowl. Peel and grate the apples, pouring away any excess juice, and add to the dried fruit. Add all the seasonings and mix. Add the 2 eggs and mix again to blend all the ingredients. At this stage the stuffing may look too sloppy – don't worry as the eggs will bind it during the cooking.

Remove the turkey from its packaging and untruss. Remove giblets, etc., from the neck and leg-end cavities. Place a small amount of butter in the base of a roasting dish which is large enough to hold the turkey easily but not too large. Roast vegetables must be cooked in a separate dish. Place the turkey in the dish and push the stuffing into both ends of the bird, folding down the flap of skin at the neck end to hold the stuffing in, and pinning the leg end with cocktail sticks. Sprinkle all over with garlic granules. Place slices of butter all over the breast and legs. Arrange the bay leaves and rosemary over the breast. Cover loosely with foil and put in a slow oven 150°C (300°F, gas mark 2) for 4 hours.

After the first hour, remove the foil and baste. Do not replace the foil. Baste at least every hour throughout. Roast vegetables should be cooked on a rack above the turkey after the first hour. Add several tablespoons of pan drippings from the turkey to the vegetables. If you are not cooking roast vegetables, keep an eye on the turkey – if it appears to brown too much, the foil should be replaced.

Before serving, remove the turkey from the roasting dish and keep warm. The pan drippings in the roasting dish will contain browned bits of stuffing that has oozed out during the cooking, which help to make a delicious gravy. Tilt the roasting dish, skim off as much fat as possible, replace over a low heat, scrape up the brownings and blend into the pan drippings. You don't need to add anything more to the gravy – it's delicious as it is – but if you want to increase the quantity, add any of the following: about 225 ml (8 fl oz) of water or either red or white wine, a teaspoon of honey-mustard, a tablespoon or so of Greek yoghurt, crème fraîche or cream.

Bring the gravy to the boil and reduce slightly, stirring well. The gravy will appear slightly lumpy because of the stuffing bits. If you can't stand this, pour into blender and blend until smooth. Reheat and serve.

Pork

Pork with fruit (lactose-free)

Ingredients   **Serves four**

    4 pork chops
    6 stoned prunes
    12 dried apricots
    2 sweet apples
    1–2 teaspoons garlic granules
    1 teaspoon dried mixed herbs
    1 teaspoon Heinz tomato sauce (or any other starch-free ketchup)
    wine glass white wine or water
    salt
    oil for frying

Method

Remove all unwanted fat from the chops and sprinkle with the garlic granules. Heat a small amount of oil in a frying pan and brown the chops on each side. Remove them from the heat. Place the chops in an oven-proof dish.

Chop the prunes and apricots. Peel and grate the apples. Mix the fruit together and layer it over the chops. Return the pan to a low heat and add the tomato sauce and water or wine. Stir, scraping the brownings from the pan and blend. Add a pinch of salt.

Pour the sauce over the chops and fruit. Cover with lid or foil and cook in a moderate oven at 180°C (350°F or gas mark 4) for 1–1½ hours.

Loin of pork with milk

Ingredients   **Serves six**

    2 kg (4 lb) loin of pork
    75 g (3 oz) butter
    1 litre (2 pints) milk
    salt

Method

No pork crackling with this dish – the excess fat should be trimmed off and the pork should be boned. Dust the meat with salt and allow to stand for 30 minutes or so at room temperature.

Melt the butter in a deep, heavy cooking pan with a lid (Dutch oven). Place the meat in the pan and fry on all sides until golden brown. Add the milk, cover the pan and cook slowly over a moderate heat for about 2 hours or until meat is thoroughly cooked. The milk sauce will be creamy and thick and slightly brown in colour.

Remove the meat from the pan, place it on a serving dish and keep warm. If desired, a teaspoon of garlic granules can be stirred into the milk sauce. Allow it to cook for a few minutes and serve with the meat.

Afelia (lactose-free)

This is a favourite dish of well-known Greek chef Sotos Achilleos.

Ingredients
about 225 g (8 oz) per person of pork fillet or boned loin or shoulder (if making for a large number, other ingredients may need to be increased)
enough dry red wine to nearly cover the meat
3 cloves garlic
1 teaspoon onion granules
1 tablespoon lemon juice
1 tablespoon honey
handful crushed coriander seeds
salt to taste
olive oil
Greek yoghurt

Method
The correct Greek way of cooking this dish is to leave the fat on the meat. Of course, you must please yourself – if you're worried about cholesterol, cut the fat off. Cut the pork into chunky cubes. Place in a glass, china or stainless-steel bowl – not aluminium.

Crush the garlic roughly – don't purée it – and add it to the wine with all the other ingredients. Stir to blend and pour over the meat. Marinate overnight.

Heat the olive oil over a medium heat. Remove the meat from the marinade with a slotted spoon, place in a frying pan with a lid and cook covered until the meat is browned and tender, stirring frequently. For the last 5 minutes of the cooking time, turn the heat low and toss the meat in the frying pan with lid on – Sotos swears this helps to tenderise the meat. Serve.

Sauce (optional)

Drain marinade to remove garlic. Return a cup or so of the drained marinade to the frying pan and stir into the meat brownings. Add a couple of tablespoons Greek yoghurt and stir to blend. Serve with the meat.

Pork fillet with orange

Ingredients

Serves four

725 g (1½ lb) pork fillet
garlic granules
75 g (3 oz) butter
150 ml (¼ pint) orange juice
1 fresh orange
4 tablespoons orange liqueur

Method

Remove any excess fat or gristle from the pork and slice it into inch-thick (2–3 cm) rounds and sprinkle lightly with garlic granules. Thinly peel the skin of the orange with a potato peeler, being careful to get only the orange zest and none of the bitter white pith, and cut into very fine matchstick strips. Squeeze the orange and add the juice to the 150 ml (¼ pint) of orange juice.

Melt the butter in a frying pan and add the pork, frying 2–3 minutes on each side. Remove the pork to a warm plate. Add the orange juice to the pan and simmer for a few minutes. Add the orange sticks and the orange liqueur. Simmer until the sauce begins to thicken. Return the pork to the pan, along with any juices, and continue to cook for one more minute. Serve with the sauce.

Pork and peach meatballs (lactose-free)

Makes 9 balls. I often make twice the recipe as this dish freezes very well.

Ingredients   **Serves two to three**

    500 g (1 lb) minced pork
    1 egg
    2 teaspoons garlic granules
    1 tablespoon dried tarragon
    salt
    5 large dried ready-to-eat peaches (juicy type; apricots can be used but
       peaches are best)
    3 rashers streaky bacon, diced

Sauce

    bottle red or white wine
    1 can pitted black olives with liquid
    Dijon mustard
    fresh tomato stock (about 1 cup or 5–6 stock cubes; see index)
    dried dill
    dash runny honey (optional)

Method

Gently fry bacon in non-stick pan. Mix first 5 ingredients. Remove bacon. Place dried peaches on chopping board, open out and cut each in half. Put small amount of bacon inside each one, close up. These may open out again, but just pinch them together when you put them inside the meat. Wash hands well. Wet with cold water. Place about a dessertspoonful of pork mixture on one hand, flatten and put peach with bacon in middle. Close pork mixture around peach and mould into ball. If possible, store in refrigerator for about an hour. Fry gently in same non-stick pan over high heat, turning until brown on both sides. Remove balls and place in baking dish. These meatballs can be cooked without the sauce and eaten cold or hot in their dry state. If you wish to do this, put them in a moderate oven 180°C (350°F, gas mark 4) and cook for about 30 minutes. If you want to make a sauce, move meatballs to warm oven and make sauce in pan as follows.

    Add 2 teaspoons Dijon mustard to brownings in pan. Stir on low heat. Add enough wine to turn the pan drippings into a thin sauce. Add complete can of pitted olives with liquid and fresh tomato stock cubes, and dried dill to taste (I usually use about 2 dessertspoons). Add a knob of dairy-free spread or butter (not lactose-free). Simmer until sauce is beginning to thicken. Check seasonings. You may wish to add a dash of runny honey. Pour over meatballs and cook, covered, in moderately hot oven 220°C (400°F, gas mark 6) for about 15–20 minutes or until cooked through.

Baked gammon with mustard sauce

Ingredients **Serves four to six**

1.25 kg (2½ lb) gammon
550 ml (1 pint) cider or apple juice
1–2 tablespoons soft brown sugar

Mustard Sauce (optional)
1 egg
2 teaspoons sugar
2 teaspoons sharp Dijon mustard
4 tablespoons malt or white vinegar
1 cup liquid meat is cooked in
1 tablespoon Greek yoghurt or double cream
salt and pepper to taste

Method
Soak the gammon for 24 hours in cold water in the fridge. Drain and put it into a pan. Cover it with water again, bring to the boil and boil for 12 minutes. Remove from the heat and drain. Place the meat in a deep oven-proof dish, pour the cider or apple juice around it and bake for 1–1¼ hours in a moderate oven at 180°C (350°F or gas mark 4), basting with the juice. Take the meat from the oven, remove the skin but not the fat. Allow it to cool slightly then press sugar into the fat. Return to the oven for 30 minutes.

To make the mustard sauce, break the egg into a small saucepan, stir in the sugar, the Dijon mustard and the vinegar. Begin to stir over a very low heat, slowly adding a cup of liquid from the meat, until the sauce begins to thicken. Stir in the yoghurt or cream and simmer until desired consistency is achieved. Adjust the seasonings. Remove the meat from the oven and serve with the sauce.

Pork and pears

Ingredients   **Serves two**

   2 loin pork chops
   2 tablespoons olive oil
   salt
   garlic granules
   2 ripe peeled pears cut into slices
   225 ml (8 fl oz) apple juice
   1 tablespoon plain mild yoghurt

Method

Sprinkle the chops with garlic granules, then heat the oil in a frying
pan and add the chops. Cook over a high heat on both sides to seal the
meat. Turn the heat down, add the pears and cook for about 10–15
minutes until tender and browned. Move the chops and pears on to a
warm plate. Pour any excess fat from the pan, return to the heat and
add the apple juice. Scrape the brownings into the juice and stir well.
Simmer until reduced by about half. Add the yoghurt and stir to blend.
Add salt to taste. Pour over the chops and serve.

Pork with Marsala (lactose-free)

Ingredients   **Serves four**

   725 g (1½ lb) pork fillet
   3 tablespoons olive or sunflower oil
   salt
   100 ml (4 fl oz) Marsala wine

Method

Slice the pork fillet into inch-thick (2–3 cm) medallion slices, heat the
oil in a frying pan and brown quickly on both sides. Sprinkle with salt,
then pour in the Marsala. Lower the heat a little and cook for a few
minutes until the meat is cooked through and the liquid reduced.

Pork chops and apple crumble

Ingredients   **Serves two**
    2 loin pork chops
    2 teaspoons garlic granules
    25 g (1 oz) butter
    1 tablespoon cooking oil
    2 sweet eating apples such as Gala
    150 ml (¼ pint) apple juice or cider or white wine
    1 teaspoon honey-mustard
    75 g (3 oz) ground almonds
    *125 g (4 oz) mild cooking cheese – Cheddar, Emmental, Gruyère or
        Jarlsburg, etc.*

Method
Sprinkle the chops with garlic powder on both sides, melt the butter
and oil together in a frying pan and fry the chops until lightly browned
on both sides. Remove from the heat and place the chops in a single
layer in an oven-proof dish.

Peel and slice each cooking apple into eight slices. Return the pan to
the heat and quickly brown apples on both sides in the pan juices.
Remove the pan from the heat and layer the apples over the chops.

Return the pan to a low heat, add the honey-mustard and juice or
cider or wine. Stir well to blend the pan brownings. Pour over the
apples and chops. Cover and cook in a moderate oven at 180°C (350°F
or gas mark 4) for 45 minutes.

Meanwhile, grate the cheese and mix with the ground almonds.
Take the chops from the oven, uncover and pour the cheese and
almond mixture over. Return to the oven and cook for a further 15
minutes or until the top is brown and the cheese bubbling.

Beef

The best roasting beef will have a marbling of fat through the meat. This gives it a wonderful flavour and keeps it tender. This can also be cooked at a higher heat for a shorter time.

Best roast beef (lactose-free)

Slow roasting beef until rare or just medium is better for today's lean cuts of meat to ensure juicier, more tender results. For topside or silverside, set the oven to 140°C (275°F, gas mark 1) and cook for about 40 minutes per pound or 90 minutes per kilogram. However, the shape of a roast may cause variation in cooking time. A rolled, tied roast may be thicker and take an extra 10 minutes per pound (500 grams). Usually, instead of sprinkling the roast with flour, I sprinkle with dried garlic granules and sometimes coat with Dijon coarse-grain mustard.

Ingredients   **Serves eight**

2.5 kg (5 lb) joint of beef (topside or top rump)
50 g (2 oz) dairy-free spread
1 tablespoon Dijon mustard, either grain or smooth
2–3 teaspoons smooth Dijon mustard
250 ml (8 fl oz) of water
wineglass of wine – either red or white
garlic granules

Method
Pat meat dry and place in a large roasting tin. Sprinkle with garlic granules. Mix the dairy-free spread and the mustard together and spread evenly over the meat. Place in a hot oven 230°C (450°F or gas mark 8) and cook for 20 minutes. Turn the oven temperature down to 180°C (350°F or gas mark 4) and roast for a further 25–30 minutes per kg (60–75 minutes) for medium beef depending on the thickness of the joint. Remove meat, stand in a warm place and cover with foil while making the gravy. Tilt the roasting dish, allow the fat to rise to the surface and skim it off with a large flat spoon, leaving the pan juices. There may not be much fat, depending on the fattiness of the beef. Pour about a cup of water into the pan and place on the stove. Add the smooth Dijon mustard and stir into the juices, scraping the browning from the sides and bottom of the pan. When all begins to thicken, add the wine and taste. You may wish to add more wine or water. Simmer until reaching the right consistency. Serve in a gravy boat.

Hamburgers galore

Basic ingredients   **Serves two**

225 g (8 oz) minced beef – not too lean, as this makes the burger too dry
salt to taste
25 g (1 oz) butter
1 tablespoon cooking oil

Method

Mix beef with a sprinkling of salt and mould into two patties. Heat the butter and oil in a frying pan. When sizzling, fry the burgers on both sides until crisp and springy to the touch – 3–4 minutes for rare burgers, longer for well done. Remove from the heat, keep warm. At this stage you can make a sauce by adding a couple of tablespoons of water or wine to the pan drippings and a teaspoon or two of Dijon mustard, to serve over the burgers.

Add these variations to the minced beef basic recipe:

- 2 tablespoons each of grated cheese and chopped parsley.
- A lump of blue cheese about the size of a walnut, stuffed in the middle of the burger.
- A tablespoon cream mixed with ½ teaspoon of garlic granules.
- 2 teaspoons mild Dijon mustard.
- 2 teaspoons dried herbs and a squeeze of lemon juice.

Fillet steak with garlic pepper (lactose-free)

The most important hint I can offer about cooking steak is to buy the best steak you can afford. Nothing can replace quality – no amount of marinating or fancy sauces will really replace the wonderful texture and flavour of a quality steak. The best fillet has tiny threads of fat running through the meat, although with the present attitude to cholesterol, it is becoming harder and harder to find. Fillet steak is now very competitively priced by comparison with lamb, and you can eat almost every morsel, so it is not the extravagance it once was. Very simple cooking will suffice to do justice to a good fillet steak. This recipe includes fresh garlic slivers in the steak, imparting a delicate garlicky aroma through the meat.

Ingredients

thickish steak per person – at least 3–5 cm (1½–2 inches) thick
clove of garlic

garlic-infused olive oil
garlic granules
red wine (optional)

Method

Trim the steaks of any unnecessary fat or sinew. Peel the garlic and slice into slivers. Make small cuts in each steak and slip a sliver of garlic into each. Place a heavy-based frying pan or grill over a high heat for a minute to so, until very hot. Rub a small dribble of garlic-infused oil on to one side of each steak. Place steaks oil-side down in the pan and cook on a high heat, turning once. Pour a little oil on to the other side before turning. For a rare steak cook 5–6 minutes each side. For medium, 7–8 minutes each side. Well done, 10–12 minutes each side. This depends on the thickness of the steak. If you are unsure, test by piercing with a sharp knife and seeing how 'bloody' it is inside. Remove the steak just before you think the colour inside is about right. Place the steaks on a warm plate and de-glaze the pan juices with a slosh of red wine if you wish – this is entirely optional. You can also add a little mustard or salt to taste, or you can simply serve the steaks without anything else.

Fillet in the piece with creamy mustard sauce

You will need half a whole fillet and it doesn't really matter which end of the fillet you choose – ask your butcher to advise you.

Ingredients   Serves six
½ a whole beef fillet
2–3 cloves garlic
about 4 teaspoons garlic granules
2–3 tablespoons mild whole-seed or Dijon mustard
100–225 ml (4–8 fl oz) red wine
1 teaspoon extra mustard
2–3 tablespoons cream (optional)
125 g (4 oz) butter or dairy-free spread

Method

Trim the fillet of surplus fat, gristle or sinew, especially the tough silvery layer along the top, which should be carefully 'skinned' off, using a very sharp knife: slide the blade of the knife under the skin and pull towards you, cutting as close to the skin as possible. Peel the garlic cloves and slice into thin slivers. Stud the fillet with the slivers of garlic by making slits all over with the point of a sharp knife and inserting a sliver into each.

In a small bowl, blend the butter/spread, about 2 teaspoons of the garlic granules and the mustard. Sprinkle one side of the fillet with garlic granules and spread with the mustard, butter/garlic mixture. Turn into roasting dish butter-side down and repeat so that the fillet is completely covered, including the ends.

Place in a hot oven 230°C (450°F, gas mark 8) for 5 minutes. Reduce the heat to 180°C (350°F, gas mark 4) and cook for about 25 minutes for rare meat or longer if preferred – slip the point of a sharp knife into the middle of the fillet and see how rare it looks. Remove just before desired 'doneness' and place on a warm plate.

Tilt the roasting pan, skim off the fat, return the pan to the heat and add the extra mustard and wine. Stir into the pan drippings and boil for a few seconds. Add cream if desired and serve with the fillet, which may be sliced thinly like roast beef or in thick 'fillet mignon' sized pieces.

Carpet bag steaks

Steaks can be filled with oysters several hours ahead and kept covered in a refrigerator.

Ingredients   **Serves four**
    16 oysters
    1 tablespoon lemon juice
    4 thick fillet steaks
    50 g (2 oz) melted buter
    100 ml (4 fl oz) red wine
    2 teaspoons Dijon wholegrain mustard
    25 g (1 oz) extra butter

Method
Combine the oysters and lemon juice in a small bowl and marinate for at least 15 minutes. Cut a small pocket in the side of each steak and fill with the oysters. Secure the openings with cocktail sticks. Brush the steaks with butter and cook in a frying pan over a high heat, turning frequently and brushing with more butter during cooking, until cooked as desired.

Remove the steaks to a warm plate. Pour the wine into the pan, scrape the pan drippings and blend. Add the mustard and simmer for a few seconds. Add the extra butter, blend and serve over the steak.

Meatballs in soured cream sauce

Ingredients   Serves two

350 g (12 oz) minced beef
1 teaspoon onion granules
1 teaspoon garlic granules
1 tablespoon starch-free tomato ketchup
1 tablespoon wholegrain Dijon mustard
½ teaspoon Greek mustard with black olives (optional)
1 tablespoon dried mixed herbs
2 eggs
2 tablespoons oil
225 ml (8 fl oz) water or 100 ml (4 fl oz) wine and 100 ml (4 fl oz) water
    or 225 ml (8 fl oz) apple juice
1 teaspoon honey-mustard
100 ml (4 fl oz) soured cream
salt and pepper

Method

Combine the first eight ingredients and mix well. Shape into smallish balls, place on a plate in a single layer and refrigerate for 30 minutes. Heat the oil in a frying pan over a medium heat, add the meatballs and cook gently until well browned all over and cooked through. Do not cover during cooking as this will make the meatballs fall apart. Remove from the pan and keep warm.

Pour any excess fat or oil from the pan. Return to the heat. Add the water/wine/juice and scrape down the pan brownings. Add the honey-mustard and bring to the boil and reduce a little. Stir in the soured cream, blend well, adjust the seasonings and return the meatballs to sauce. Simmer uncovered until heated through. Serve.

Beef cacciatore

I have included several recipes made with tomatoes but before you decide to try them, read my notes about tomatoes at the beginning of the soups section, page 104. This recipe makes a wonderful sauce for Bolognaise, lasagne or cacciatore, which is a pot-roast. Pot-roasting is another name for braising, and is ideal for chuck steak or blade steak as better cuts tend to become too dry. But it's not always easy to get chuck steak or blade steak in a large piece, and the magic of a pot-roast is being able to carve the meat, dripping in delicious savoury juices, while serving the sauce separately. I have often used silverside when unable to get a solid piece of braising steak.

Ingredients

1.5 kg (3 lb) piece of beef – braising steak or silverside
2 tablespoons oil
2–3 fresh bay leaves
3–4 tablespoons dried onion granules
3 teaspoons garlic granules
300 ml (½ pint) dry red or white wine
1½ tablespoons vinegar
300 ml (½ pint) water
100 ml (4 fl oz) jellied chicken stock (optional)
1 teaspoon dried basil
1 tablespoon dried mixed Italian/Mediterranean herbs
1–2 teaspoons sugar
75 g (3 oz) butter or dairy-free spread
500 g (1 lb) fresh peeled tomatoes or 450 ml (16 fl oz) tomato juice
3 anchovy fillets
2 tablespoons milk
50 g (2 oz) stoned black olives
1 tablespoon chopped parsley

Method

Trim the surplus fat off the meat. Heat the oil in a large deep oven-proof dish or 'Dutch oven'. Add the meat and brown on all sides. Remove the meat and set aside. Return the pan to the heat. Slosh in the vinegar and bay leaves, then very quickly add the wine. Boil until reduced by half, then add the water and the chicken stock and stir over the heat for about 2 minutes.

Blend or sieve the tomatoes if necessary, and pour into the pan. Add the onions, garlic granules, herbs and sugar, then boil all together for a few moments, stirring well. Add the butter and stir until blended, then taste the mixture. If you think it needs more salt or sugar, add at this stage.

Return the meat to the pan, cover and cook in a moderate oven at 180°C (350°F or gas mark 4) for 1 to 1½ hours until tender. Meanwhile, soak the anchovy fillets in milk and cut the olives in half. Remove the meat and stand on a warm plate. Drain the anchovies, chop them finely and add to the sauce, with the olives and parsley. Reheat and simmer for a minute. At this stage the meat can be returned to the sauce to await serving – just stand over a very low heat so that it is just keeping warm.

Carve the meat and serve the sauce separately. Serve with noodles or mashed potato for the family or visitors.

Lasagne

This is a way of making proper lasagne for the rest of the family and a small mock lasagne for yourself in a separate dish. You will need a Bolognaise sauce made either from your own recipe or use the recipe for beef cacciatore, substituting 1.5 kg (3 lb) of mince instead of the braising steak. You can either make half the recipe or make up the whole amount, and freeze half for another occasion. Both the sauce and the finished lasagne freeze well. If you want a less rich sauce, omit the anchovies and olives and add more water.

Ingredients   **Serves three to four**
Bolognaise sauce made with 750 g (1½ lb) mince
1 packet dried lasagne pasta, spinach or plain, or same amount fresh
750 g (1½ lb) cottage cheese
2 eggs
2 tablespoons chopped parsley
75 g (3 oz) grated Parmesan cheese
225 g (8 oz) mild grated cheese
2 teaspoons salt

Method
Have ready a large oblong lasagne dish and a small oven-proof dish for yourself. Lightly butter both dishes.

In a large mixing bowl beat the eggs, add the cottage cheese and blend well. Mix in the Parmesan cheese, parsley and 1 cup of mild grated cheese. Add salt to taste.

Place a layer of lasagne on the bottom of the large dish – if you are using dried pasta, dip the strips in a dish of warm water before layering. Spread a layer of meat sauce over, then a layer of cottage cheese sauce, then repeat with pasta, meat sauce and cottage cheese, finishing with cottage cheese.

Leave enough meat and cheese sauce for yourself. Spread the desired amount of meat sauce in the small dish and top with cottage cheese. Sprinkle the remaining grated cheese over both dishes. Cook in a moderate oven at 180°C (350°F or gas mark 4) until bubbling and beginning to brown on top. Serve with a salad.

Lamb

Old-fashioned roast lamb with real mint sauce (lactose-free)

Ingredients   **Serves four to six**

1 good-sized leg of lamb – at least 2¼ kg (4½ lb)
several cloves of garlic
several sprigs fresh rosemary (optional)
garlic granules to sprinkle
beef dripping or lard or a mixture of olive oil and dairy-free spread

Method

The lamb should be completely covered with a thin layer of fat, which is necessary to keep in the juices. Wipe and pat dry. With a sharp knife, slice the ends off the garlic cloves, slip the skins off and slice each one into several slim slivers. Make deep slits all over the lamb with the point of the knife, inserting the garlic as you go, and a leaf or so of the rosemary. Dust the leg with garlic granules.

Melt the dripping, lard or oil and spread in a roasting tin to cover the bottom. Place the lamb in the tin, tilt the tin so that the fat runs to one side and baste the lamb thinly with the fat. Place in a slow to moderate oven (150°C–180°C, 300°F–350°F, gas mark 2–4) and roast for 30–35 minutes to the pound (500 g) – over two hours. This will produce an old-fashioned well-done roast. If you want a modern slightly rarer roast, cook in a moderate oven for 20 minutes to the pound (500 g) with 20 minutes over. Baste the meat several times during the cooking. A roasting bag can be used but this tends to braise the meat, rather than roast it.

Real mint sauce

Pick enough fresh mint to make 3–4 tablespoons when chopped. Wash the mint well, shake dry and strip the leaves. Discard the stalks, place the leaves on a chopping board and sprinkle with a tablespoon of ordinary granulated sugar. Begin to chop with a large sharp knife – the size of a carving knife. Hold the tip of the blade in one hand and the handle of the knife in the other, and chop up and down, scraping the mint into the centre again as it rolls out to the edge.

Sprinkle with another tablespoon of sugar and keep chopping until the mint is very fine and pulpy. Scrape into a serving jug and barely cover with boiling water and about 100 ml (4 fl oz) of vinegar – either white or malt. Stir a few times and leave to steep. Serve with the lamb.

Glazed leg of lamb (lactose-free)

Guaranteed to produce a deliciously tender roast with wonderful flavour and a marvellous gravy.

Quince jam is the best for this recipe, but is not always readily available. Do not use jelly jam, as it is too slippery to coat the lamb properly and slides off. The jam glaze does not produce a particularly sweet flavour, as you might think, but acts as a tenderising marinade.

Ingredients   **Serves eight**

1 large leg of lamb
1 or 2 jars best redcurrant, quince or apricot jam
two cloves garlic (optional)
olive oil

Method
Line a roasting tin with sheets of foil, making sure there are no slits in the foil so that the meat and jam juices cannot escape into the roasting tin during the cooking. Lightly oil the foil base. If using garlic, remove skins and slice into slivers. Make deep slits all over the lamb with the point of a knife, inserting the garlic as you go. Score the top of the lamb lightly with a diamond pattern. Spread with the jam, place in the foil and wrap around. Bake in a moderate oven 180°C (350°F or gas mark 4) for about 2½ hours, basting occasionally during the cooking.

Unwrap the foil, spread some more jam over the meat and bake for a further 30–45 minutes, uncovered. Remove the meat to a warm serving plate. Carefully lift the foil from the roasting tin, pouring all the juices back into the tin. Discard the foil. Tilt the tin and allow the fat to rise to the top. Skim the fat off with a large spoon. Place the tin over a low heat and simmer until the juices are reduced. You will not need to add anything extra to this gravy. If you think it needs diluting, you could add water and perhaps a little cream, but it is best just as it comes. The joint is equally delicious hot or cold.

Des Britten's lamb (lactose-free)

Ingredients   **Serves four**

whole loin of lamb, boned, including fillet
several sprigs of fresh rosemary
1–2 teaspoons garlic granules
25 g (1 oz) dairy-free spread
3 tablespoons redcurrant jelly
1 teaspoon mild Dijon mustard

Method

Ask the butcher to bone the lamb for you or do it yourself: first cut off the fillet, then with a sharp knife slice down inside of the bones along the loin. Discard the bones, fat and skin.

Pull the rosemary leaves off their sprigs and chop roughly. Spread the loin open, lie the fillet in the middle, brush with dairy-free spread, then sprinkle with rosemary and garlic granules. Roll up the lamb and tie with string.

Cook in an open roasting dish or oven-proof dish in a moderate oven at 180°C (350°F or gas mark 4) for 40–50 minutes or until cooked as desired. Turn off the oven and leave for about 10 minutes.

In a small saucepan mix the redcurrant jelly with the mustard and heat together. Slice the lamb into thick 'fillet mignon' sized pieces and spoon the sauce over the meat.

Marinated lamb chops (lactose-free)

Ingredients   **Serves two to three**

   6 lamb chops
   65 ml (2½ fl oz) raspberry vinegar
   2 tablespoons redcurrant or cranberry jelly
   1 tablespoon fresh rosemary
   150 ml (about ¼ pint) extra-virgin olive oil
   2 tablespoons fresh orange juice

Method

Trim lamb chops of fat. Place in bowl. Wash rosemary and pull the small leaves off the woody stem. Whisk together with remaining ingredients until combined. Pour marinade over chops and leave for at least an hour – if marinating in the fridge, leave for several hours. Remove chops from marinade and cook in oven or over barbecue, until done. The chops will be very tender but if cooking in oven a sheet of roasting film on top helps to keep them moist.

Everyday meals

Quick, easy and economical for lunch or supper.

Bacon star

Ingredients   **Serves two**
  750 g (1½ lb) bacon rashers
  1–2 sweet apples, depending on size
  175 g (6 oz) mild cheese – Emmental, Gruyère, Jarlsburg, Cheddar –
    whatever you prefer as long as it's mild

Method
Lay the bacon rashers in a large shallow oven-proof dish and put it in
a hot oven at 200°C (400°F or gas mark 6). I use a large quiche dish and
arrange the bacon in a cartwheel design. Peel and grate the apple.
Grate the cheese. Remove the partly cooked bacon from the oven and
cover with a layer of apple and top with the grated cheese. Return to
the oven and cook until the cheese is melted and beginning to brown –
about 20 minutes. This can be eaten as a cold savoury, sliced into
fingers. It is very handy for taking as a snack when travelling.

Simple braised steak

Ingredients   **Serves four to five**
  1 kg (2 lb) chuck steak
  2 tablespoons dried onion granules
  1 teaspoon garlic granules
  salt
  100 ml (4 fl oz) claret or water
  1 tablespoon chopped parsley (optional)

Method
Trim any gristle or fat from the steak and cut into serving size pieces.
Mix the dried onions and garlic granules together on a dinner plate
and press the steak on to the mixture, turning and coating each side
liberally. Place in a casserole dish and sprinkle any remaining dried
vegetables over the meat. Season with salt to taste. Pour the water or
claret over and cover the casserole with a lid or tightly with foil. Bake
in a moderate oven at 180°C (350°F or gas mark 4) for 1½ hours or until
tender.
    Don't be tempted to add more liquid in the initial stages of cooking
– the meat juices and the dried onions combine together with the small
amount of liquid to form a luscious gravy.

Grandma's rissoles

Ingredients   **Serves four**
about 500 g (1 lb) leftover roast beef
2 eggs
4 tablespoons chopped parsley
2 teaspoons Dijon mustard
1 tablespoon non-starch vinaigrette dressing
1 tablespoon Heinz tomato sauce
1 tablespoon dried onion granules

Method
Mince the beef, add the other ingredients and mix well, or process everything in a food processor, adding the beef first and chopping roughly, then the other ingredients. Spoon into patty tins and cook in a moderate oven at 180°C (350°F or gas mark 4) for about 30 minutes.

Alternatively, squeeze small handfuls together, roll in a mixture of ground almonds and garlic powder and fry in hot oil until brown.

Frankfurter sauté

Ingredients   **Serves two to three**
10 pack Herta skinless frankfurters (or any starch-free frankfurters)
1 tablespoon dried onions
1 sweet apple
3 tablespoons Greek yoghurt
1 tablespoon cooking oil
2 teaspoons Heinz tomato ketchup
2 teaspoons Dijon mustard

Method
Cube the frankfurters. Peel, core and cube the apples. Heat the oil in a frying pan over a medium heat, add onions and sauté for 2 minutes. Add the apples and sauté for two minutes. Add the frankfurters and lightly brown. Mix the yoghurt with the tomato ketchup and mustard. Pour over the frankfurters and cook over a low heat, stirring occasionally until the sauce is brown and thick. Serve.

Quick gammon bake

Ingredients   Serves one

1 large thick slice cooked gammon or ham
1 teaspoon mild sweet Dijon or any starch-free mustard
1 small eating apple
1–2 slices cheese

Method

Spread the mustard over the ham. Peel and slice the apple. Lay it over the ham, then place the cheese over the apple. Grill or cook in a hot oven at 200°C (400°F or gas mark 6) until the cheese is brown and bubbling.

Cheese and bacon cream

Ingredients   Serves one

125 g (4 oz) medium Cheddar or Swiss-type cheese, grated
250 ml (8 fl oz) whipping cream
1 egg beaten
2 rashers bacon

Method

Dice and fry the bacon gently until cooked but not crisp. Combine with the other ingredients and pour into a buttered oven-proof dish. Bake in a moderate oven at 180°C (350°F or gas mark 4) for 20 minutes.

Spicy haddock steaks

Ingredients   Serves one

1–2 haddock steaks, fresh or defrosted from frozen
25 g (1 oz) butter or dairy-free spread
1 tablespoon lemon juice
2 teaspoons Heinz or any starch-free tomato ketchup
1 teaspoon mild Dijon mustard

Sauce

½ clove crushed garlic
1 teaspoon mild Dijon mustard
150 g (5 oz) mild low-fat yoghurt

Method

In a small saucepan, melt the butter, then add the lemon juice, tomato ketchup and mustard. Heat through gently – don't worry if the mixture curdles. Remove from the heat.

Brush the fish steaks with the mixture on one side. Cook under a hot grill or in a hot oven at 200°C (400°F or gas mark 6) for about 5 minutes. Remove from the heat, turn and brush the other side of the fish with the mixture. Continue cooking for another 5 minutes. Meanwhile, blend the garlic, mustard and yoghurt. Serve sauce cold with fish.

Frittata

Ingredients   Serves four
6 eggs
4 tablespoons onion granules
400 g (14 oz) whole peeled tomatoes
25 g (1 oz) butter
1 tablespoon cooking oil
3 slices ham
1 tablespoon chopped parsley
½ teaspoon fresh or dried basil
2 tablespoons grated Parmesan cheese

Method
Chop the tomatoes roughly. Finely chop the ham, parsley and basil, and combine in a large bowl with the tomatoes, onions and Parmesan cheese. Whisk the eggs, then pour over the tomato mixture and blend well.

Melt the butter and oil together in a shallow pan. Pour in the mixture and cook over a very low heat for about 10 minutes, without stirring. Place the pan under a hot grill or in a hot oven at 200°C (400°F or gas mark 6) until the mixture is set. Do not let the top brown. Cut into wedges and serve with a salad. This can also be eaten cold.

Puffed cheese fish

Ingredients   Serves three to four
6 medium fillets white fish
salt
2–3 tablespoons cooking oil
100 ml (4 fl oz) starch-free mayonnaise
125 g (4 oz) grated mild–medium Cheddar
1 tablespoon chopped parsley
1 teaspoon lemon juice
1 stiffly beaten egg white

Method
Wash and dry the fish, sprinkle with salt and lightly brown on both sides in the cooking oil. Remove from the heat, drain and lay the fish in a buttered oven-proof dish. Combine the remaining ingredients and pile over the fish fillets. Bake in a moderate oven at 180°C (350°F or gas mark 4) for 12 minutes or until the coating is puffed and browned.

Tomato cheesy scrambled eggs for one

Ingredients
  2 eggs
  25 g (1 oz) butter
  75 ml (2½ fl oz) milk (approximately)
  handful grated cheese
  pinch salt
  1 beefsteak tomato, sliced thickly

Method
Beat the eggs with a fork, then add the milk and salt. Melt the butter in a frying pan over a low heat and pour in the eggs. Cook very slowly, until just beginning to set. Throw the cheese on to the eggs and cook a few more seconds until set. Remove from the heat, then pile the eggs on to the sliced tomatoes and eat.

Tomato and cottage cheese salad for one

Ingredients
  1 large beefsteak tomato
  small pack of cottage cheese
  ½ teaspoon sugar
  ½ teaspoon garlic granules
  starch-free steak seasoning or mixed herbs

Method
Cut the tomato in half. Sprinkle each half with the sugar, salt and garlic granules. Pile the cottage cheese on to each half and sprinkle with a little steak seasoning. Chopped chives may also be added.

Baked apple savoury (lactose-free)

Ingredients   **Serves one**

    1 large sweet apple
    1 Herta frankfurter
    2 teaspoons dairy-free spread
    1 teaspoon sweet Dijon mustard
    dash Heinz tomato ketchup

Method

Core the apple to make a hole big enough to insert the frankfurter. Beat the butter, mustard and ketchup together. Spread on top of the apple. Cook in a hot oven until tender.

Egg and spinach casserole

Ingredients   **Serves four**

    1 kg (2 lb) spinach
    75 g (3 oz) butter
    2–3 eggs, beaten
    2–3 tablespoons grated Parmesan cheese
    chopped marjoram (optional)
    salt

Method

Pile the spinach into a sink full of water, stir and dunk in the water until all leaves are washed, then leave to soak while the sand sinks to the bottom. Remove the spinach, change the water and repeat the process three times in all. This is very important as spinach is grown in sand. It is also the reason pre-washed spinach is so much dearer – and I think worth paying for!

Pile the leaves into a large saucepan, press down well, put the lid on and cook unsalted and without additional water for 2–3 minutes or until tender. Remove from the heat, put a plate into the saucepan, hold over the sink and press the plate down, draining the water away. Get the spinach as well drained as possible.

Melt the butter in an oven-proof casserole dish, add the spinach and season lightly with salt. Mix the beaten eggs with the Parmesan cheese and the marjoram, pour over the spinach, stir to blend and place in a hot oven at 200°C (400°F or gas mark 6) until the eggs are set.

Swedish beef olives

Ingredients

Serves two

350 g (12 oz) thinly sliced beef – topside, rump or chuck
2 large sweet apples
12 finely chopped dried apricots
6 chopped stoned prunes
2 tablespoons chopped parsley
2 teaspoons mixed dried herbs
1 tablespoon finely chopped pitted green olives (optional)
2 eggs
salt
25 g (1 oz) butter
1 tablespoon oil for cooking
2 teaspoons honey-mustard
100 ml (4 fl oz) water
wine glass of wine – red or white
2 tablespoons mild plain yoghurt

Method

You can buy thin slices of beef for beef olives in most supermarkets, but if you have to prepare it yourself, buy as lean a piece of meat as possible, and slice thinly with a very sharp knife into rectangles which will roll up when stuffed into cylinders the size of small sausages. Then beat the beef with the edge of a saucer or a meat mallet until as thin as possible, without making holes in the meat.

Peel and grate the apples and mix with the finely chopped dried fruit, herbs, parsley and olives. Beat the eggs and add to the fruit mixture. Season with salt to taste. Combine until well blended.

Put spoonfuls of mixture on each slice of beef and roll up. Secure with cocktail sticks or tie with string. Brown quickly on each side in a frying pan. Remove from the heat and place in a single layer in an oven-proof dish. Return the pan to the heat, add the honey-mustard, water, wine and yoghurt, and stir well to blend. Remove from the heat and pour over the beef olives. Cook in slow oven at 140°C (275°F or gas mark 1) for 1½ hours or until tender. They can be cooked in a very low oven or slow cooker for 3–4 hours.

Pork pockets (lactose-free)

Ingredients **Serves four**

    4 good large thick pork chops or steaks
    sprinkle of garlic granules
    oil for frying
    stuffing as for Swedish beef olives (see previous recipe)
    350 ml (12 fl oz) orange juice

Method

Slice through the chops or steaks to create a pocket. Stuff with the stuffing. If necessary, seal the edge with cocktail sticks. Lightly sprinkle garlic granules over one side of the meat and brown quickly, garlic side down, in oil in the frying pan. Sprinkle garlic granules over the upper side and turn to brown. Remove the pan from the heat and place the meat in a single layer in an oven-proof dish. Return the pan to the heat, pour in the orange juice and stir with the pan brownings, boil to reduce slightly and pour over the meat. Cook in a moderate oven at 180°C (350°F or gas mark 4) for 1–1½ hours or until tender.

Gammon Jonathan

Ingredients **Serves one to two**

    1 large slice of ham or gammon – about 3 cm (1½ inches) thick
    25 g (1 oz) butter
    1 tablespoon brown sugar
    1 teaspoon strong Dijon mustard
    small carton cream

Method

Melt the butter in a frying pan and fry the ham lightly on both sides. Mix the mustard and sugar. Remove the ham, spread on one side with half the mustard mixture. Pour a little of the cream into a shallow oven-proof dish and place the ham, mustard side down, in this. Spread the remaining mustard mixture on the top side of the ham, then pour more cream over to cover. Lay foil over the top to cover lightly. Bake in a moderate oven at 180°C (350°F or gas mark 4) until very tender – about 45 minutes to an hour.

Fish patties with lemon sauce (lactose-free)

Ingredients   **Serves two**

750 g (1½ lb) white fish fillets
1 mild-tasting apple
1 egg
2 tablespoons chopped fresh chives
1 tablespoon fresh basil
1 tablespoon lemon juice
2 tablespoons cranberry or redcurrant jelly
1 teaspoon mild Dijon mustard
oil for greasing patty tins

Sauce

½ cup starch-free mayonnaise
2 tablespoons chopped fresh chives
1 tablespoon lemon juice

Method

Skin and bone the fish fillets. Peel and core the apple. Either finely chop the fish, grate apple then mix with the other ingredients or process until fine but not mushy. Grease 8 patty tins (put a drop of oil into the bottom of each and rub around with greaseproof paper) and press spoonfuls of the fish mixture into each patty tin and cook in a moderate oven at 180°C (350°F or gas mark 4) for about 45 minutes or until the top is beginning to brown.

Meanwhile, blend the mayonnaise, chives and lemon juice. Serve the patties with the sauce.

Scrambled sausage cups

Ingredients   **Serves one**

2 eggs
65 ml (2½ fl oz) milk
75 g (3 oz) butter
salt
2–3 slices of German garlic sausage or mild salami or other starch-free sausage
1 large tomato

Method

Beat the eggs lightly with the milk. Season with salt. Melt two-thirds of the butter in a heavy pan set on a very low heat. Pour in the egg mixture and cook covered, very slowly. Use a heat mat underneath if possible, to prevent browning on bottom.

Meanwhile, cook the sausage in a separate pan in the remainder of the butter until the edges curl up and become cup-shaped. Slice the tomato. When the eggs are cooked, place the sausage on a warmed plate, pile the eggs into each sausage cup and top with the sliced tomato.

Anzac omelette

Ingredients   **Serves one**
   2 eggs
   100 g (3½ oz) tin smoked oysters
   25 g (1 oz) butter
   2 tablespoons milk or cream

Method
Drain the oysters, then rinse and chop them roughly. Separate the eggs. Beat the whites until stiff. Mix the yolks with the milk or cream and add the chopped oysters. Fold the whites into the mixture. Melt the butter in a frying pan or omelette pan, pile the mixture into the pan and cook without stirring until almost set. Brown under a grill. Fold in half and serve.

Baked supper savoury

Ingredients
   2 eggs per person
   approximately 75 g (3 oz) cheese per person
   milk or cream
   butter
   salt

Method
Butter an oven-proof dish well and line the bottom and sides with grated cheese. Break in the eggs, pour the cream or milk over, and season with salt. Either top with more grated cheese or bake uncovered in a hot oven at 190°C (375°F or gas mark 5) for 15–20 minutes.

Denver ham patties

Ingredients   **Serves one**
  1 cup minced leftover ham
  12 g (½ oz or about 2 teaspoons) melted butter
  2 tablespoons cranberry or redcurrant jelly
  1 tablespoon chopped parsley
  1 beaten egg

Method
For each person blend one portion of the ingredients. Press the
mixture into greased patty tins (about two to three patties per
person). Set the tins in a large dish of hot water, in a hot oven at 190°C
(375°F or gas mark 5). Cook for 15–20 minutes, or until set. This can
also be made with leftover turkey but will need salt added to the
mixture to taste.

Alternative cheese bake

Ingredients   **Serves two**
  German sausage or frankfurters
  3 eggs
  250 g (9 oz) mild grated cheese
  450 ml (¾ pint) milk
  salt
  further 125 g (4 oz) grated cheese

Method
Slice the sausage or frankfurters and line a shallow buttered oven-
proof dish with the slices. Combine the next three ingredients, season
with salt to taste and pour over the sausage. Sprinkle the extra cheese
over, stand the dish in a larger dish of water, place in a moderate oven
at 180°C (350°F or gas mark 4) and bake until set (about 20–30 minutes).

Pizza omelette (lactose-free)

This must be cooked in a non-stick pan. Choose the right size, depending on how many people you are cooking for. It should be about the thickness of a pizza when cooked.

Ingredients (per person)
2 eggs
1 rasher of bacon or slice of ham
1 medium tomato
generous pinch of dried chives
salt
1 teaspoon dairy-free spread
1 tablespoon grated cheese (optional; not lactose-free)

Method
Dice the bacon or ham. Melt the dairy-free spread over a low heat in the bottom of a frying pan and scatter the bacon/ham over the bottom. Cook gently while beating the eggs with a sprinkling of salt. Pour the eggs over the bacon/ham. If you can eat dairy foods, add the cheese now. Slice the tomato thinly. When the egg mixture is beginning to thicken, arrange the tomatoes on top and sprinkle generously with dried chives. Remove pan to the oven or place underneath a medium grill until completely cooked.

Salads

I eat at least one salad every day. Raw vegetables and fruit are the best source of fibre – and besides, I love them. You really have to eat lots of salads on the IBS Low-Starch Diet so if you've always thought of salads as simply a couple of lettuce leaves and a tasteless tomato, think again. Learn to seek out the freshest and best-tasting vegetables. Don't buy when they're flabby and stale for the simple reason that they don't taste good.

Nowadays there are lovely sweet tomatoes and crisp, sweet red peppers in the shops all year round. There's a huge variety of lettuce and herbs available – be adventurous, try things you're not familiar with.

If you've steered clear of real vinaigrettes for years because of the extra calories, now you can begin enjoying them again with a clear conscience. On the low-starch diet you need the oil to compensate for the lack of the butter or margarine you used to eat on or with bread and cakes.

Olive oil is especially high in the healthy polyunsaturated fats which we are all urged to eat more of. It is also particularly noted for its purity, which means that it doesn't need to be chemically purified, unlike most other oils, which go through a number of refining processes including neutralising with caustic soda, 'washing and drying', bleaching and deodorising. I wholeheartedly recommend cold pressed virgin olive oil (first pressing) for its delicious flavour, both in cooking and in salad dressings. There are many varieties now available.

If you want to use ready-made vinaigrettes (and I often do) look for those which don't contain modified starch. It used to be difficult to find these but I'm glad to say that more and more manufacturers are using non-starch thickeners, or even traditional recipes with no additional thickening. The range is extending all the time, and the quality is very good.

Store salad carefully and it will stay fresh for longer

When you're making salad frequently you need a variety of ingredients to offset possible boredom. And if you're making it only for yourself, it's a problem to get through them before they go stale. Correct storage is important. Most lettuces are wrapped or sold in plastic bags these days. When you begin to use it, remove the lettuce from the wrapping, discard the outer leaves, remove the leaves you plan to use and wash well. Don't wash the rest of the lettuce at this stage unless it is very dirty, as this will slightly damage the leaves and cause lettuce 'rust' and slime. Don't put it back in the original wrapper as this may be dirty. Store in a fresh plastic bag in your refrigerator. Sprinkle a little water into the bag on the leaves and they should keep well for almost a week.

Store tomatoes, peppers, radishes and cucumbers unwashed and leave any stalks on until just before use. Store celery and carrots unwashed, but do discard tough outer celery stalks. The other half of an onion stores well for a couple of days in the refrigerator, covered in food-wrap.

Some herbs such as parsley store better after washing, but they must be drained well and stored in a plastic bag. Herbs with delicate leaves, such as rocket and basil, tend to wilt quickly, but don't react well to a rough washing. Don't disturb them unless they're looking very jaded. Use them soon after buying or buy in the pots and water as instructed.

Mushrooms are best left undisturbed in their original packs. Buy small amounts, remove those you want to use and return the rest to the fridge. Brown paper bags are often recommended for mushrooms, but I honestly don't think it makes any difference.

Bags of pre-washed mixed salad are more expensive and don't last as well, but save space in your refrigerator.

Simple green salad (lactose-free)

I never get tired of a mixture of greens and herbs with a good dressing. Best made every day but you can make enough for two days and store the rest without dressing in a bowl, covered with cling-wrap, in the fridge.

Ingredients
> at least two different types of leaf: cos (romaine), iceberg (crisphead), little gem, bronze, oakleaf, lollo rosso, endive, Chinese cabbage, chicory or spinach
>
> at least two different types of herbs: parsley, chives, rocket, watercress, mustard and cress, lamb's lettuce, dandelion

Method
Select for a variety of colour and shape. Wash the lettuce leaves, tear into bite-sized pieces or use whole. Wash the herbs and chop if necessary. Place in a large, wider bowl than looks necessary and just before serving, add a dribble of good dressing and toss. This is really all you need, but I often add sliced mushrooms and several whole small tomatoes. The salad should look very leafy, with at most, only a few other additions for variety.

Simple coleslaw

I prefer to slice the cabbage because it has a milder taste, but some experts say the cabbage should be shredded, then soaked in ice-water for a few minutes, drained thoroughly and chilled. However you do it, a coleslaw can be as simple as:

Ingredients   **Serves four**
  approximately 275 g (10 oz) finely shredded cabbage
  100 ml (4 fl oz) any starch-free mayonnaise
  1 tablespoon cream
  salt

Method
Place cabbage in a salad bowl, sprinkle with a little salt, combine the mayonnaise with the cream and add little by little, tossing all the while. Just moisten cabbage – you may not need to use all the dressing.

To this basic recipe any or all of the following may be added. (Measurements are approximate only – use your own judgement.)

  1 cup grated carrot
  1 cup cut-up red apple with skin on
  ½ cup diced celery
  ½ cup diced red pepper
  ½ cup chopped parsley
  ½ cup chopped chives
  ½ cup diced dates

Grilled goat's cheese salad

The fresher the goat's cheese is, the milder it will be. My preference is for a mild, creamy taste, but it's entirely a matter of opinion.

Ingredients
  1 goat's cheese about 10 cm (4 inches) thick for each person
  green salad made from any combination of lettuce and herbs,
    including whole cherry tomatoes
  black olives
  capers
  vinaigrette

Method

Make the salad and arrange in a large, shallow salad bowl. Add the black olives and capers to taste. Toss with just enough vinaigrette to moisten the lettuce – don't use too much. Place the cheeses under grill or in a very hot oven, until they are beginning to brown on top and ooze tantalisingly. Remove the cheeses, arrange on the salad bowl and serve. Salads can be served in individual dishes, each topped with a goat's cheese.

Van Styvesant koolslaa

This salad was brought to New York by the Dutch settlers in 1624.

Ingredients   **Serves six**

500 g (16 oz) finely shredded white cabbage
4 tablespoons light malt vinegar (or any mild vinegar)
1 tablespoon sugar
1 teaspoon Dijon mustard
1 tablespoon butter
1 egg
2 tablespoons cream

Method

Place the cabbage in a bowl. In a separate bowl, lightly beat egg. Heat the vinegar, sugar, mustard and butter in a saucepan over a low heat, until boiling. Add some of the hot mixture to the egg, mix well then stir back into the vinegar mixture. Cook stirring until the mixture thickens and boils. Remove from the heat. Stir in the cream and pour while still hot over the cabbage. Toss. Chill and serve cold.

Onion salad (lactose-free)

Ingredients   **Serves two to three**

1 small red onion
1 small Spanish onion
1 red pepper
4 spring onions
16 pitted Spanish olives
2 tablespoons wine vinegar
65 ml (2½ fl oz) extra-virgin olive oil
2 teaspoons anchovy paste

Method
Peel and cut the onions and pepper into slices and place in a serving bowl. Peel and dice the spring onions. Chill. Place the vinegar, oil and anchovy paste in a bowl and beat vigorously. Drain the olives and arrange on the salad. Pour the dressing over and serve.

Chicken almond salad

Ingredients   **Serves four**

  350 g (12 oz) diced cooked chicken
  175 g (6 oz) raisins
  50 g (2 oz) blanched almonds
  2 tablespoons chopped parsley
  3 tablespoons diced spring onions
  1 tablespoon lemon juice
  2 tablespoons Hellman's real (or any starch-free) mayonnaise
  150 ml (¼ pint) cream
  lettuce leaves

Method
Soften the raisins in a little cold water, bring to the boil and stand for 5 minutes. Strain and cool. Combine with the chicken, almonds, parsley and spring onion. Mix the lemon juice into the mayonnaise and add the cream. Pour over the chicken mixture and toss to blend. Place spoonfuls on lettuce leaves and serve.

Salad niçoise (lactose-free)

Ingredients   **Serves four**

  6 or 8 crisp lettuce leaves
  6 ripe medium-sized tomatoes
  3 hard-boiled eggs
  500 g (1 lb) can tuna
  6 anchovy fillets
  16 black olives
  4 tablespoons virgin olive oil
  1 tablespoon wine vinegar
  1 clove garlic
  2 tablespoons chopped fresh parsley
  1 teaspoon capers
  salt

Method

Place the lettuce leaves whole in a bowl, unless they are very large, in which case tear them in half. Cut the tomatoes and eggs into quarters. Roughly flake the tuna. Add all to the lettuce leaves.

Peel the garlic and crush with the blade of a heavy knife, sprinkling salt on the garlic and crushing several times. Rinse the capers. Pour the olive oil and vinegar into a screwtop jar. Add the garlic, capers and parsley. Shake until blended. Pour over the salad and toss lightly. Place in individual dishes, scatter the olives over and lay the anchovy fillets on top.

Roast beef and asparagus salad

Ingredients   **Serves two to three**

225 g (8 oz) leftover rare roast beef
225 g (8 oz) cooked, cold, fresh asparagus (not canned)
2 small (200 g/7 oz) raw courgettes
250 g (9 oz) punnet cherry tomatoes, halved
1 or 2 little gem lettuces

Dressing

4 tablespoons plain yoghurt
1½ tablespoons starch-free tomato ketchup
1 teaspoon mild smooth Dijon mustard

Method

Slice the beef into strips. Wash the lettuce leaves and leave whole. Peel the courgettes and slice into long thin strips. Combine the beef, asparagus, courgettes, tomatoes and lettuce. Combine the dressing ingredients and pour over the salad before serving.

Watercress salad with egg dressing (lactose-free)

Ingredients   **Serves four**

3 bunches watercress
4 hard-boiled eggs
1½ tablespoons wine vinegar
¾ teaspoon salt
1 tablespoon Dijon mustard
4 tablespoons safflower oil
3 tablespoons olive oil
2 tablespoons non-starch mayonnaise

Method

Wash and dry the watercress and remove the heavy stems. Place in a large bowl. Finely chop the eggs. In a screw-top jar, combine the vinegar, salt, mustard and oils. Shake to combine. Pour into a small bowl, then add the mayonnaise and half the chopped eggs. Blend and pour enough of this mixture over the watercress to coat well. Toss. Sprinkle the remaining eggs over. Serve.

Tanya's courgette salad

Ingredients   Serves two to three

500 g (1 lb) young courgettes
2 tablespoons olive oil
salt
5–6 tablespoons Greek yoghurt
2 tablespoons roughly chopped basil leaves

Method

Wash and grate the courgettes, unpeeled. Heat the oil in a frying pan and add the courgettes. Sprinkle with salt and toss in the oil until just warmed through. Mix the basil into the yoghurt. Place the courgettes in a serving dish and pour the yoghurt over.

Aussie red heart salad (lactose-free)

Ingredients   Serves eight

½ red cabbage, sliced finely
1 packet best-quality dried apricots
6 spring onions
salt
450 ml (15 fl oz) virgin olive oil
1 clove garlic
150 ml (¼ pint) balsamic vinegar
1 teaspoon Dijon coarse-grain mustard

Method

Place the cabbage in a shallow salad bowl and arrange the apricots on top. Chop the spring onions and scatter over. Lightly season with salt. Peel the garlic and crush with the blade of a knife, sprinkling with salt. Combine all the dressing ingredients in a screw-top jar, add the garlic and shake well. Pour the dressing over the salad and allow it to stand for about 30 minutes. Toss just before serving.

Unbelievably simple salad

Ingredients
2 large or 3 medium sweet tomatoes per person
2 teaspoons chopped chives per person
2 tablespoons cream per person
salt

Method
Wash the tomatoes and slice thinly. Place on a large serving plate. Add the chopped chives to the cream, season with the salt and spoon over the tomatoes.

Greek salad

In Greece they call this the 'village salad' – *choriàtiki salàta*.

Ingredients   **Serves six**
3 large firm tomatoes
1 large cucumber
1 medium onion
2 green peppers
1 cup black olives
225 g (8 oz) feta cheese
handful each of finely chopped basil and parsley
100 ml (4 fl oz) virgin olive oil
4 tablespoons malt vinegar
1 clove garlic, crushed
salt

Method
Cut the tomatoes into chunks, slice the onions and green peppers. Peel the cucumber if the skin is tough, otherwise slice or cube. Place in a salad bowl, lightly sprinkle with salt and toss gently. Cube the feta cheese and add to the bowl with the olives and herbs. Peel and crush the garlic with the blade of a knife, sprinkling with salt and crushing several times. Pour the oil and vinegar into a screw-top jar, add the garlic, shake vigorously and pour over the salad. Toss gently again and serve.

Spinach, anchovy and egg salad (lactose-free)

Ingredients   Serves four

    enough raw spinach for four
    4 hard-boiled eggs
    8 anchovy fillets
    4 tablespoons of your favourite dressing or this recipe:
        6 tablespoons virgin olive oil
        2 tablespoons white wine vinegar
        1 clove garlic

Method

Wash the spinach thoroughly, remove the stems, shake dry and drain in a colander. If the leaves are large, break them into bite-sized pieces and arrange in a salad bowl. Drain the anchovy fillets, cut into quarters and add to the spinach.

Make a dressing by blending the oil and vinegar in a screw-top jar. Peel and crush the garlic sprinkled with salt with the blade of a knife, then add to the jar and shake vigorously.

Cut two of the eggs into quarters and chop the other two finely. Just before serving, pour the dressing over the spinach and toss. Sprinkle the chopped eggs over and arrange the quartered eggs around the edge of the bowl.

Spinach and bacon with blue cheese dressing

Ingredients   Serves four

    80 g (3 oz) (2–3) streaky bacon rashers
    enough raw spinach for four
    3 hard-boiled eggs
    bunch of chives
    225 g (8 oz) sweet cherry tomatoes

Dressing

    1 tablespoon sugar
    1 teaspoon salt
    1 teaspoon Dijon mustard
    3 tablespoons wine vinegar
    150 ml (¼ pint) salad oil
    125 g (4 oz) Roquefort or Danish blue cheese

Method

Dice the bacon and cook over a very low heat until crisp – don't let it burn. Drain. Wash the spinach well, drain and if the leaves are large, tear them into bite-sized pieces. Put in a salad bowl. Wash the tomatoes, chop the chives and add to the salad with the bacon. Toss lightly.

Combine all the dressing ingredients, except the cheese, in a screw-top jar and shake until blended. In a separate bowl, mash the cheese and add enough dressing to make it sufficiently pourable (about half a cup). Pour over the salad and toss lightly. Chop the eggs finely and scatter over the salad. Left-over dressing can be used in other salads.

Tomato and anchovy salad (lactose-free)

Ingredients   Serves four

6–8 medium sweet tomatoes
2 teaspoons salt
1 bunch chives
6 fresh basil leaves
45 g (approx. 2 oz) tin anchovies in oil

Dressing

150 ml (¼ pint) virgin olive oil
4 cloves garlic
3 tablespoons white wine vinegar or sherry vinegar
pinch sugar
salt

Method

Make the vinaigrette first: peel the garlic, sprinkle with salt and crush under the blade of a strong knife. Sprinkle with salt and crush several times. Combine the oil and vinegar in a screw-top jar, add the garlic and sugar. Shake vigorously and allow to stand for several hours.

Place the tomatoes in a bowl and pour boiling water over them. After a few seconds spear each one with a fork and peel off the skin. Slice the tomatoes thickly, place in a colander and sprinkle with salt. Leave to drain for about an hour. Arrange on a serving dish.

Chop the herbs, open the tin of anchovies and drain. Spoon the vinaigrette over the tomatoes, sprinkle the herbs over and lay anchovies in a lattice pattern on top. Serve.

Salmon salad (lactose-free)

This salad can be a complete meal.

Ingredients   **Serves one to two**
  1 or 2 little gem lettuces
  3 sticks celery
  1 large firm tomato
  ½ red pepper
  ½ yellow pepper
  1 tablespoon chopped parsley
  213 g (approx. 8 oz) can pink salmon
  vinaigrette dressing of your choice

Method
Wash all the vegetables. Separate the leaves of the lettuce, break into
bite-sized pieces and put in a serving bowl. Chop the celery, slice the
red and yellow peppers into strips, cut the tomato into segments, chop
the parsley and add them all to the lettuce. Pour a little dressing over
the vegetables and toss. Add the salmon and toss lightly again. Serve.

Chicken salad (lactose-free)

Ingredients   **Serves two**
  a variety of greens such as: 2 leaves iceberg lettuce, 2 leaves lollo rosso, 2
      little gem lettuces or 4–5 leaves cos lettuce
  handful rocket leaves
  handful spinach
  1 tablespoon chopped chives
  1 tablespoon chopped parsley
  6 sliced mushrooms
  about a dozen whole cherry tomatoes
  2 cold breasts of Slimmers' Simple Chicken cooked in foil (see index)

Method
Wash and break the lettuce leaves into bite-sized pieces and place in a
salad bowl. Wash the tomatoes, chop the herbs and mushrooms, and
add to the bowl. Chop the chicken into strips or cubes, add to the bowl
and pour your favourite vinaigrette dressing over, or use your own
mayonnaise.

Cucumber salad Damascus

Cool and refreshing. Try this with rich meat dishes.

Ingredients **Serves two**
    1 cucumber
    2 tablespoons plain yoghurt
    ½ clove garlic
    2 tablespoons chopped chives
    1 tablespoon chopped mint
    salt

Method
Peel the cucumbers, slice thinly and place in a mixing bowl. Peel and crush the garlic, chop the chives and mint and add to the yoghurt. Season to taste. Pour over the cucumbers and toss together.

American salad (lactose-free)

The Americans love salads made with fruit. They often serve them before the main course, but this is a wonderful summer salad served with ham or gammon.

Ingredients **Serves two to three**
    whole lettuce leaves
    2 fresh peaches
    4 halved canned pears
    20 fresh cherries
    1 small or ½ large cucumber
    4 tablespoons vinaigrette

Method
Peel the cucumber and slice thinly. Slice the pears, peel the peaches and slice by cutting into the stone all around the peach until the segments fall off (like a chocolate orange). Cut the cherries in half and remove stones. Combine all in a salad bowl, then toss in the vinaigrette. Serve in lettuce 'cups' on individual plates.

American 'jello' salads (lactose-free)

The first time I was invited to dinner with American friends and saw fruit salad in jelly on the table, I assumed it was for dessert. To my surprise, it was part of the main course. I discovered it is delicious with meat – and why not? After all, we enjoy redcurrant or mint jelly with lamb – a 'jello' salad is just a more imaginative version. The fruit used can be fresh or canned and should be well drained. A tablespoon of lemon juice or any mild vinegar can be added if desired. Leftover juice can be added to the liquid required for the jelly. Fresh, uncooked pineapple and kiwi fruit will prevent the jelly from setting. Canned pineapple is fine, but kiwi fruit is best used only as a garnish. Here are two versions.

Version one ingredients
1 lime jelly
about 350 g (12 oz) sliced pears, apricots and sweet green grapes

Version two ingredients
1 orange jelly
about 350 g (12 oz) orange segments and strawberries

Method
Make the jelly according to the directions, then add the fruit. Set either in a jelly mould, individual moulds or an ordinary deep dish. Brush the mould with light salad oil before pouring the liquid jelly in. Chill until firm. Unmould and serve on a bed of lettuce or garnished with watercress or parsley.

Warm garlic tomato salad

Ingredients   **Serves one to two**
1 box sweet cherry tomatoes
75 g (3 oz) butter
1 teaspoon garlic granules
salt

Method
Melt the butter in a frying pan over a low heat. Add the garlic granules and heat but do not brown. Add the tomatoes. Heat for 4 minutes over a very low heat, sprinkle with salt to taste. Serve hot on a bed of lettuce or watercress.

Warm mushroom salad (lactose-free)

Ingredients **Serves four**

150 g (5 oz) pack of small button mushrooms
8 cloves of garlic or 1 solo garlic
1 tablespoon or more extra-virgin olive oil
2 teaspoons dried herbes de Provence or Italian herbs
2 little gem lettuces
vinaigrette

Method
Wash and dry the mushrooms and remove stalks. Wash and dry the lettuce and place in a salad bowl. Peel the garlic, and if using solo garlic, cut into eighths. Pour the oil into a frying pan, add the garlic and cook gently until the garlic begins to infuse the oil. Don't allow to get too brown. Add the mushrooms and toss in the oil. Lastly, sprinkle the herbs over. Cook lightly until the mushrooms are well warmed through but not mushy. Remove from heat and spoon on to the lettuce. Drizzle with vinaigrette and serve.

Puddings and desserts

Spiced apricot compôte (lactose-free)

This is best made in a slow cooker, the bottom oven of an Aga or in an ordinary oven on very low heat, 85°C (180°F) for 8 hours or overnight. If you have a gas cooker, use the lowest setting (¼ or ½ or S) and put the dish on the base plate, overnight. It can also be cooked for 4 hours in a moderate oven at 170°C (325°F, gas mark 3). It is wonderful served with plain Greek yoghurt or vanilla ice-cream.

Ingredients   **Serves four to six**

   275 g (10 oz) dried apricots
   150 ml (¼ pint) sweet white wine or sherry
   450 ml (¾ pint) water
   25 g (1 oz) sugar
   2 tablespoons mild-flavoured honey
   1 large orange, finely grated zest and juice
   1 teaspoon whole cloves

Method
Put the apricots in a flame-proof casserole, pour in the wine and water, then stir in the sugar and honey. Heat gently until dissolved, then bring to the boil. Remove from the heat, add the orange zest and juice and the cloves. Cover the casserole and cook slowly as above. Cool and remove the cloves before serving.

Brandied prune mousse

Ingredients   **Serves six**

   225 g (8 oz) stoneless prunes
   water to cover prunes
   2 tablespoons sugar
   4 tablespoons reserved prune liquid
   2 egg whites
   100 ml (4 fl oz) cream
   1 tablespoon brandy

Method
Cover the prunes with water and soak overnight. Bring to the boil, add the sugar and simmer for 15 minutes. Drain, reserving liquid, and allow to cool. Purée the prunes in a liquidiser with 4 tablespoons of the

reserved liquid or push through a sieve and add the liquid. Place in a large basin. Stir in the brandy. In a smaller basin whip the egg whites until stiff. Whip the cream separately. Fold the cream into the prune mixture and gently fold in the egg whites. Place in a serving dish and chill.

Creamy lemon freeze

Ingredients   **Serves six**
  125 g (4 oz) ground almonds
  75 g (3 oz) butter
  1–2 tablespoons sugar
  2 separated eggs
  397 g tin full-cream sweetened condensed milk
  85 ml (3 fl oz) lemon juice
  ½ teaspoon grated lemon zest
  3 tablespoons caster sugar

Method
Melt the butter over a low heat. Add the ground almonds and cook gently until they begin to brown. Remove from the heat, stir in the sugar to combine well and press into an oblong plastic food box, or loaf tin, and place in the freezer.

Beat the egg yolks until thick. Combine with the condensed milk, juice and peel. Beat the egg whites with caster sugar into a stiff meringue. Fold into the lemon mixture.

Remove the ground almonds from the freezer, pour the lemon mixture over the almond base and freeze.

Apple soufflé

Ingredients
Serves two

2 large Bramley apples or 500 g (1 lb) apple purée
125 g (4 oz) caster sugar
3 eggs
150 ml (¼ pint) crème fraîche
1 tablespoon Calvados

Method
If using fresh apples, peel, slice and cook them in a little water until soft enough to give a thick purée. Separate the eggs, whisk the whites until stiff and set them aside. Beat the yolks, sugar, Calvados and crème fraîche until thick and add the apple. Blend well. Fold in the egg whites, pour into a greased soufflé dish and bake in preheated oven (180°C, 350°F, gas mark 4) for 50–60 minutes or until just set. Serve hot or warm with cream.

Choc-orange mousse

Easy to make with a blender or food processor.

Ingredients
Serves eight

300 ml (½ pint) cream
225 g (8 oz) plain (dark) chocolate
2 tablespoons sugar
4 egg yolks
1 tablespoon Grand Marnier
1 teaspoon vanilla
2 teaspoons grated orange zest
50 g (2 oz) unsalted butter

Optional topping
1 whole orange
200 ml (7 fl oz) water
125 g (4 oz) sugar
120 ml (4 fl oz) whipping cream
2 teaspoons Grand Marnier

Method
Break or chop the chocolate and place it, with the butter, in the top of a double boiler or in a bowl set into a saucepan, a quarter filled with

water (do not let the bowl touch the bottom). Melt together over simmering water. Add 300 ml (½ pint) cream to the chocolate mixture and heat slowly, stirring, until bubbles form around edges (do not boil), then remove from the heat.

Meanwhile, grate the orange zest and place in a food blender with the egg yolks, sugar and Grand Marnier. Begin to blend the egg mixture on low speed while pouring in the hot chololate/cream mixture, then blend all together on high speed for about a minute or until smooth. Pour into 8 small serving glasses. Refrigerate 1 to 2 hours before serving. Serve with whipped cream or topping.

For the topping, peel the rind thinly from the orange or use a zester, and boil for 5 minutes in plain water. Drain and cut into thread-like strips. Combine the water and sugar, bring to the boil, add the orange rind and cook until rind is transparent (about 4 minutes). Remove and cool. Beat the cream and Grand Marnier until thick. Pipe or blob spoonfuls of cream on the serving dishes with the orange rind twirled on top.

Superb cheesecake

Most shop-bought cheesecakes include cornflour or flour, but there's no need. This is an absolutely brilliant recipe – however, a word of warning about the cream cheese. I have discovered that the Philadelphia brand, when tested with iodine, goes a strange olive-greenish colour, indicating there may be starchy additions not listed on the pack. Plain unbranded cream cheese from the deli counter of your supermarket or food store is fine.

Ingredients   Serves eight
750 g (1 lb 8 oz) unbranded cream cheese – not low-fat
75 g (3 oz) caster sugar
125 g (4 oz) mild-flavoured honey
5 large eggs
100 ml (4 fl oz) thick soured cream
100 ml (4 fl oz) thick plain cream
1½ teaspoons freshly grated lemon zest
65 ml (2½ fl oz) lemon juice
½ teaspoon salt

Method
Prepare a 24 cm (9½ inch) diameter round spring-form cake tin by buttering all over the sides and bottom and sprinkling with icing sugar (make sure the icing sugar is starch-free). Shake upside-down over the

sink to remove surplus sugar. Or, alternatively, line an ordinary cake tin with baking parchment – cut a circle for the bottom and strips for the side. If you wish, this can be made in a loaf tin or casserole dish, but whatever you use, it must be properly prepared so that cheesecake can be turned out easily.

In a large bowl, beat the cream cheese with an electric beater until light and fluffy, adding the sugar and honey gradually, and beating until well combined. Add the eggs one at a time, then both creams, vanilla essence, lemon zest, juice and salt. Pour the mixture into the prepared tin and bake in a moderate oven (170°C–180°C, 350°F, gas mark 4) for 1 hour. Check the cake – if the top is getting too brown, lay a sheet of baking parchment or brown paper on top. If the cake springs back leaving no fingerprint when it is touched in the middle, it is ready. Turn off the oven, open the oven door and leave to cool.

Refrigerate overnight. Turn out on to a serving plate the next day. Serve with whole strawberries covered with strawberry sauce. This may require a longer cooking time – I cooked it for 2 hours in a loaf tin.

Key-lime mousse

One of the most popular desserts in America is key-lime pie. Here is an adapted version – just as delicious without the pie crust. Key-limes are an American variety unobtainable here, so this is not really key-lime anything. Ordinary limes will do just as well.

Ingredients   **Serves four to six**
   1 envelope unflavoured gelatine
   120 ml (4 fl oz) fresh lime juice
   125 g (4 oz) sugar
   125 g (4 oz) mild-flavoured honey
   2 large eggs, beaten
   175 g (6 oz) natural full-cream cream cheese (unbranded)
   175 g (6 oz) butter, softened
   500 ml (18 fl oz) whipping cream, divided into two parts
   1½ teaspoons grated lime zest

Method
Wash the limes, grate the zest and set aside. Squeeze the juice and pour it into a medium-sized saucepan. Sprinkle the gelatine over the juice and allow to stand for 5 minutes. Beat the eggs and add with the sugar and honey to the juice. Stir with a wooden spoon or wire whisk until blended. Cook over a medium heat, stirring constantly, until the

mixture comes to the boil. Reduce the heat and simmer, stirring constantly, for about 3 minutes or until thickened. Remove from the heat and set aside.

Beat the cream cheese and butter with an electric beater until smooth. Gradually add the lime juice mixture, beating well. Cover and chill for 25 minutes, stirring occasionally.

Beat 250 ml (9 fl oz) of whipping cream until stiff peaks form. Fold into the chilled lime mixture. Cover and chill for a further 25 minutes, stirring occasionally.

Beat the remaining cream until stiff peaks form. Fold into the chilled mixture with the grated zest. Pour into individual dishes if desired. Cover and chill for 4 hours or until firm.

Strawberry and yoghurt sorbet

Ingredients   **Serves four**
   125 g (4 oz) sugar
   150 ml (¼ pint) water
   250 g (9 oz) strawberries
   225 ml (8 fl oz) plain mild low-fat yoghurt
   1 egg white

Method
Combine the sugar and water in a saucepan, stir constantly over heat without boiling until the sugar is dissolved. Bring to the boil, reduce the heat, simmer uncovered without stirring for five minutes or until the mixture is thick. Cool the sugar syrup to room temperature and refrigerate until cold.

Blend or process the strawberries and yoghurt until smooth, add the sugar syrup and blend. Pour mixture into a pie dish or oblong plastic food container or similar, cover with foil and freeze for several hours or until set.

Beat the egg white until stiff, remove the frozen mixture, break it up with a fork, beat until smooth and fold in the egg white. Return to the container and freeze again until set. This can be made three days ahead and kept covered in the freezer.

Brandied figs

Ingredients   Serves three
12 fresh figs
250 ml (8 fl oz) brandy
75 g (3 oz) sugar
125 g (4 oz) honey
thick cream or Greek yoghurt

Method
Peel the figs and place in a bowl. Dissolve the sugar and honey in the
brandy, pour over the figs and chill in the refrigerator for several hours
or overnight. Turn the figs occasionally to make sure all are well
soaked in the brandy. Serve with cream or Greek yoghurt.

Baked apple slices (lactose-free)

Ingredients   Serves two
500 g (1 lb) Bramley apples
2 tablespoons sugar
about 50 g (2 oz) dairy-free spread or butter (not lactose-free)
piece of lemon zest (optional)

Method
Peel, core and slice the apples and place in a single layer in a shallow
oven-proof dish. Sprinkle the sugar over evenly, cut the spread into
small pieces and dot all over (you may need a little more). Wash a
lemon and carefully peel a slice off the skin, making sure you get only
the zest and none of the bitter white pith underneath. Place the peel in
the centre of the dish and cook, uncovered, and without any water, in
the top of a medium oven for about 30 minutes. Check that all the slices
are cooking evenly from time to time, and turn them over halfway
through the cooking. Delicious hot or cold, with ice-cream, custard or
cream, or as the filling for a sweet puffy omelette.

In cider
Omit the lemon peel and spread. Pour in some cider up to two-thirds
the height of the apples and cook as above.

In orange juice
Use orange juice and grated orange peel instead of cider.

Sweet puffy omelette (lactose-free)

Ingredients
Serves two to three

3 eggs
2 tablespoons caster sugar
a sherry glass of any sweet liqueur such as Grand Marnier, Cointreau,
    kirsch, cherry brandy, apricot brandy or rum
25 g (1 oz) butter or dairy-free spread

Method
Preheat the oven to a moderate heat (180°C, 350°F, gas mark 4). Separate the eggs into two medium-sized mixing bowls. Add 1 tablespoon of sugar to the whites and beat until stiff. Add 1 tablespoon of sugar to the yolks and beat until thick and lemon-coloured. Beat in the liqueur. Fold the white mixture carefully into the yolks.

Melt the butter or spread over a high heat in a heavy frying pan with an oven-proof handle. When the butter is sizzling, pour the egg mixture in and turn the heat to low. Cook slowly until light brown underneath (about 10 minutes). Bubbles will still appear through the uncooked puffy top and the mixture will look moist. Remove the frying pan and place in the oven. Bake until the omelette is light brown on top and springs back leaving no fingerprint when lightly touched in middle (about 10–15 minutes). Remove from the oven, make a deep crease across the omelette, place any filling on one half, slip a spatula underneath to loosen, fold over and turn out on to a warm plate. Slice into wedges and if desired serve with cream. This is wonderful with strawberries marinated in orange juice, or raspberry purée.

Low-cal baked apple (lactose-free)

Ingredients
Serves one

handful sultanas or raisins
1 teaspoon runny honey
4 tablespoons unsweetened orange juice
1 large eating apple

Method
Put the dried fruit, honey and orange juice in a basin and stand for at least 10 minutes. Wash the apple well, core but do not peel, and stand in an oven-proof dish. Spoon the dried fruit into the hole, pour the juice over, cover with a lid or foil and bake in slow to moderate oven (170°C, 325°F, gas mark 3) for 45 minutes.

Custard sauce

We can't eat custard made with custard powder or cornflour, whether bought in packs or cans, on trifles or mixed with fruit or jelly. But we can eat proper custard made with eggs, bought or homemade.

Custard sauce can be made in an ordinary heavy-based saucepan if you are an experienced cook and you stir constantly with a wooden spoon to prevent the mixture from curdling. Even if curdling does occur, a lump of butter stirred in at the end will make the mixture smooth again. But all good cooks say (and I agree) that it is best made in a double boiler or a bowl fitted into a saucepan of simmering water (don't let the bottom of the bowl rest on the bottom of the saucepan). Well-made egg custard sauce is one of the great dishes of the world. Here is the recommended standard version.

Ingredients   **Serves four**

4 egg yolks or 2 whole eggs
25 g (1 oz) sugar
¼ teaspoon salt
350 ml (12 fl oz) milk
1 teaspoon vanilla essence

Method
Quarter fill a saucepan or the bottom of double boiler with water and stand over the heat to boil. Whisk the sugar, salt and eggs together until the mixture is thick and almost white. Bring the milk almost to the boil and pour through a sieve into the egg mixture, stirring at the same time. Reduce the heat under the water until it is simmering. Place the bowl (or top of double boiler) containing the egg mixture over simmering water and stir constantly. As soon as the mixture begins to coat the spoon and before it begins to boil, remove from the heat, add the vanilla and continue stirring for a couple of minutes.

Floating island custard

Ingredients   **Serves four**

　2 *egg whites*
　¼ *teaspoon salt*
　2 *tablespoons caster sugar*
　900 *ml (1½ pints) milk*

Custard sauce

　3 *whole eggs*
　2 *egg yolks*
　3 *tablespoons sugar*
　pinch salt
　1½ *teaspoon vanilla essence*
　more milk if needed

Method

Beat egg whites with salt and sugar until stiff. In large diameter saucepan or deep frying pan, bring the milk to simmer and drop rounded tablespoonfuls of egg white mixture on top. Poach gently, uncovered, in the simmering milk until firm (about 5 minutes). Remove the meringues with a spatula and set aside on a plate.

Beat whole eggs, egg yolks, sugar and salt together until thick. Measure the heated milk and add more to make up to 900 ml (1½ pints) if necessary. Pour through a sieve on to the egg mixture and place in the top of a double boiler or in a bowl in a saucepan and cook, stirring constantly, as in the custard sauce recipe. Remove from the heat, add the vanilla and continue to stir for a while. Pour into a serving bowl. Place the meringues on top. Chill and serve.

Crème anglaise

This is a deluxe version of custard sauce as made by the French and named after the English – who usually only make the standard version.

Ingredients   **Serves four**
 1 vanilla pod
 600 ml (1 pint) milk
 8 egg yolks
 75 g (3 oz) sugar
 pinch salt

Method
Split the vanilla pod in half lengthways and place in the milk. Bring to the boil and remove from the heat. Leave to infuse for 15 minutes. Whisk sugar, salt and egg yolks until the mixture is almost white. Return the milk to the heat and bring almost to the boil, pour through a sieve into the egg mixture stirring constantly, and cook in a double boiler or a bowl over simmering water as in the standard recipe – but do not add any extra vanilla at the end. Additional flavours such as kirsch, rum or brandy can be stirred into the cooled custard.

Baked custard

Ingredients   **Serves two to three**
 3 eggs
 475 ml (16 fl oz) milk
 25 g (1 oz) sugar
 pinch salt
 1 teaspoon vanilla essence

Method
Bring the milk almost to the boil, remove from the heat. Whisk the eggs, sugar and salt together until combined and pour the milk over, continuing to whisk. Add the vanilla essence and pour into a pie dish and stand this in a large pan of hot water shallow enough to come halfway up the side of the pie dish. Place in a slow oven (150°C, 300°F, gas mark 2) and bake for an hour or until a knife inserted in the custard, slightly off-centre, comes out clean. Remove and serve warm or chilled.

Crème caramel

Ingredients   **Serves six**
 5 tablespoons sugar
 150 ml (¼ pint) water
 7 eggs
 900 ml (1½ pints) milk
 120 ml (4 fl oz) cream
 1 teaspoon vanilla essence
 4 tablespoons sugar
 pinch salt

Method
In a small saucepan over a low heat, dissolve the 5 tablespoons of sugar in the water, stirring constantly. When dissolved, stop stirring and allow it to boil rapidly until it turns golden brown. Remove from the heat and pour immediately into a deep, round oven-proof dish. Quickly tilt the dish to make the caramel coat the bottom of the dish evenly. Set aside.

Lightly whisk the eggs, 4 tablespoons of sugar and salt together in a bowl. Heat the milk and cream to just under boiling, then pour this over the egg mixture, whisking continuously. Add the vanilla essence. Pour the mixture through a sieve on to the caramel mixture. Place in a large baking pan filled with enough hot water to come halfway up the side of the dish.

Bake in a slow oven (150°C, 300°F, gas mark 2) for 40 minutes to an hour, or until a knife inserted in centre comes out clean. Remove and cool to room temperature before chilling overnight.

To serve, run a knife around the inside edge to loosen, put a serving dish over the top and turn upside-down.

Crème brûlée

Ingredients   **Serves six**

  6 egg yolks
  4 tablespoons caster sugar
  900 ml (about 1½ pints) cream
  pinch salt
  2 teaspoons vanilla essence
  further caster and brown sugar

Method

Beat the egg yolks, 4 tablespoons of caster sugar and salt together until thick. Heat the cream in the top of a double boiler or a bowl set in a saucepan of simmering water until nearly boiling. Remove and pour over the eggs, stirring continuously. Stir in the vanilla and pour all through a sieve into an oven-proof dish set in a baking pan of hot water. Bake 1–1½ hours in a moderate oven (160°C, 300°F, gas mark 2) until a knife inserted into the centre comes out clean. Do not overbake – the custard will continue to cook from retained heat when it is removed from the oven. Cool and chill overnight. Before serving, cover the entire surface with a mixture of caster and brown sugar, set in a dish of ice-cubes and put under the grill until the sugar melts and browns. Allow to cool and refrigerate until topping is firm.

Peach clafouti

Ingredients   **Serves two**

  325 g (11 oz) can peach slices
  750 g (1½ lb) ricotta cheese
  2 teaspoons grated lemon zest
  2 tablespoons peach juice
  75 g (3 oz) sugar
  120 ml (4 fl oz) full-cream evaporated milk
  2 eggs

Method

Drain the peaches, saving the juice, and lay the slices on the bottom of a deep oven-proof dish. Wash the lemon carefully and grate the zest. Beat the ricotta cheese with an electric beater until fluffy. Beat in the milk, rind, peach juice, sugar and eggs. Pour over the peach slices and bake in a moderate oven at 180°C (350°F or gas mark 4) for about 50 minutes or until a knife inserted into the centre comes out clean.

This recipe can also be made with baked apple slices (see index).

Swiss cream

Ingredients   **Serves four**
  1 jelly – any flavour
  1 cup boiling water
  410 g (14 oz) (large can) full-cream evaporated milk

Method
Chill the can of milk overnight or put it in the freezer for 1½ hours.
Make up the jelly with the boiling water, according to instructions.
Leave until cool. Pour the chilled milk into a large bowl and beat with
an electric beater until thick. Pour the cooled jelly into milk and beat
again. Leave to set.

Wine jelly (lactose-free)

Ingredients   **Serves three to four**
  1 raspberry jelly
  250 ml (8 fl oz) boiling water
  250 ml (8 fl oz) red wine

Method
Make up the jelly according to the instructions with the boiling water.
Cool. Add the wine. Pour into small serving dishes and chill. Serve
with cream and summer fruits.

Orange yoghurt with raspberries

Ingredients   **Serves six**
  500 g (1 lb) carton of mild low-fat plain or Greek yoghurt
  ½ jar of orange curd – see index (if made from bought curd, make sure it is
     starch-free)
  1 carton frozen raspberries
  2 tablespoons sugar
  2 teaspoons water (optional)

Method
Put the raspberries (either frozen or defrosted) in a small saucepan and
bring slowly to the boil. You do not need to add any water unless you
prefer a less intense taste – you can always add it afterwards if you
think it is needed. Stir gently so as not to break up the fruit and when
simmering remove from the heat. Add sugar to taste, gently mixing
until it is dissolved. Chill.

Pour the yoghurt into a mixing bowl and blend with the orange curd. Use more curd if desired. Chill. Serve the raspberries in small glass bowls topped with the yoghurt.

Perfect pavlova

This is an unconventional method that really works. It makes a perfect crisp crust with soft marshmallow centre – and it does not sink when you take it out of the oven. Because it is cooked at such a low heat, it does not cause IBS symptoms unless you eat too much.

Ingredients   **Serves four to six**
  4 egg whites
  pinch salt
  225 g (8 oz) caster sugar
  1 teaspoon each of vanilla essence and white vinegar
  4 tablespoons boiling water

Method
Heat the oven to 200°C or 400°F or gas mark 6. Cut a piece of baking parchment or foil large enough to cover an oven tray. Butter well (rub all over with a lump of butter held in butter paper) and sprinkle with water.

Beat all the ingredients together with an electric mixer until it holds firm peaks when you take the beaters out of the mixture. Pile the mixture on to the prepared paper. The mixture will spread a little so make it into a rounded shape that is higher than you want the finished pavlova to be. Do not shape it with a hollow in the middle – this is not a true pavlova. Place in the oven, close the door and turn the oven off. Leave for 1½ hours or overnight. To serve, cover with cream and decorate with fruit.

To make in an Aga, put the pavlova into the roasting oven for 7 minutes. Remove to the simmering oven for 4½ hours.

It is traditional to decorate pavlovas with passionfruit or a passionfruit sauce. Unfortunately, this is one of the few fruits that contain starch (in the pips) and this is especially intense when the fruit has been cooked. So do not use passionfruit.

Zabaglione (lactose-free)

There are many recipes for zabaglione. This one uses both Marsala and dry white wine and is also delicious poured warm over ice-cream or fruit. You will need an electric egg-beater.

Ingredients   **Serves four**
5 large egg yolks
4 level tablespoons caster sugar
150 ml (5 fl oz) Marsala wine
85 ml (3 fl oz) dry white wine

Method
Have ready a large saucepan with a couple of inches of water in the bottom. This must be large enough so that the bowl in which you will beat the egg yolks can sit over the water, but not so large that the bowl touches the bottom of the saucepan or the water. Carefully separate the eggs, placing only the yolks into the bowl (you could make a large pavlova with the whites). Put the saucepan over a low heat so that the water is just simmering when you need it. Don't put the bowl into the saucepan yet. Add the sugar to the egg yolks and begin beating with the electric beater until the mixture is pale and creamy. Gradually beat in half the Marsala and half the white wine little by little, about a tablespoon at a time. Gradually beat in the remaining Marsala and wine. Transfer the bowl to the saucepan, keeping the heat very low and making sure the bowl doesn't touch the water. Continue beating until the mixture thickens and becomes foamy. This will take about 10–15 minutes, but don't be tempted to turn the heat up, because if the mixture becomes too hot it will curdle. When it is thick enough for the beaters to leave a clear trail on the top when they are lifted out of the mixture, it is ready. Serve in 4 shallow champagne glasses (or something of that size) that have been warmed beforehand.

Baking

Marie Antoinette's advice was right: 'If they can't eat bread, let them eat cake!' We can't eat bread – this is one food for which I cannot find a substitute. But I can offer some very good cakes and biscuits made without flour or starch.

Some ten years ago, when I first began experimenting with this diet, I missed cakes and pastries terribly. Now I no longer miss the comfort of these foods – I can pass even the most delicious cakes and biscuits without a second glance – but I would miss the convenience. Life is so much easier when you can snack on a biscuit or a piece of cake to keep you going.

I discovered there's virtually no such thing as a bought cake that is starch-free, so I was forced to devise my own recipes. A number of classic cakes are made with ground almonds which are quite a good substitute for the taste and texture of flour. The only trouble is that ground almonds are more expensive, make a far richer cake and one can't eat as much. However, they're very delicious and will help you feel less deprived.

If you've never done much baking before, I suggest you buy a good basic book with illustrations which show you how to prepare cake tins, test for 'doneness' – all the basic things that are not always spelled out in recipes. Baking is really rewarding and the secret is to be well organised. Read the recipe thoroughly, prepare the cake tins first and then assemble everything you need before you start mixing (as they do on TV cooking programmes).

You'll find baking paper or parchment a great boon as you won't be able to flour the cake tins. But there's a trick to using baking parchment successfully – butter or grease the tin you're going to cook in, *before* you line it with parchment, and the parchment will stick to the surface of the tin instead of slipping and sliding about.

Because oven temperatures tend to vary slightly, it is wise to test the cake for doneness yourself, rather than sticking exactly to a specific cooking time. I use two methods:

(1) Insert a heavy darning needle or fine skewer into the centre. If it comes out clean, the cake is cooked. If it still looks sticky, the cake is not ready.
(2) This method is best for light cakes. Touch the top lightly with a finger. If the fingerprint disappears, the cake is done.

It is better to remove a cake when slightly under-baked as it will carry on cooking as it stands.

I hope these starch-free cakes and biscuits will help with your withdrawal pangs.

Basic cake batter

Ingredients
75 g (3 oz) butter or dairy-free spread
75 g (3 oz) sugar
¼ teaspoon salt
3 eggs, separated
175 g (6 oz) ground almonds
1 teaspoon desired flavouring essence (optional)
sultanas, cherries, etc. (optional)

Method
This cake is not light and fluffy and will not rise greatly. It has a consistency similar to gingerbread. Prepare a cake tin with baking parchment. Beat the egg white until stiff. Cream the butter, salt, sugar, and add egg yolks. Beat until thick and creamy. Add essence and any fruit or chocolate. Add the ground almonds. Pour into the cake tin and bake in a moderate oven (180°C, 350°F, gas mark 4) for about an hour. Test after 50 minutes by inserting a large darning needle or fine skewer into the centre of the cake. If it comes out clean, the cake is cooked.

Plain cake
add 1 teaspoon of vanilla essence

Almond cake
add 1 teaspoon of almond essence (the ground almonds by themselves do not give a very almondy flavour)

Cherry cake
add 125 g (4 oz) chopped cherries and ½ teaspoon of almond essence

Sultana cake
add 175 g (6 oz) sultanas and ½ teaspoon of vanilla or rum essence

Orange cake
add grated peel of an orange and 1 teaspoon of orange essence

Basic biscuit batter

If you've ever made choux pastry, this method will be familiar to you. I cannot be absolutely precise about the amount of ground almonds because it depends a great deal on how finely they are ground. The finest are almost like flour and 'bind' better than those of a slightly coarser grind. The recipe is a successful way of making a biscuit-type batter with many uses for savoury or sweet biscuits, cheesecake and pie bases or a sort of crumbly, cakey topping for fruit puddings. Experiment with your own ideas.

Ingredients
90 ml (3½ fl oz) water
25 g (1 oz) butter
90–125 g (3–4 oz) ground almonds
2 eggs

Method
Simmer the water and butter together in a saucepan until the butter is completely melted. Remove from the heat and add the almonds – enough for the mixture to have a dense consistency. Beat in the eggs with a wooden spoon until the mixture is thick and smoothish. Cool and add any of the variations below. Blend well and place the mixture in spoonfuls or balls on a baking tray which has been prepared with baking parchment. The mixture spreads somewhat during cooking. Bake in a moderate oven (180°C, 350°F, gas mark 4) until beginning to brown.

For cheese biscuits
To the dry ground almonds add:
125 g (4 oz) grated cheese
1 teaspoon salt

Blend well and add to the water/butter mixture, before beating in the eggs. Place on a piece of baking parchment and roll into a long log. Wrap in the parchment and chill for 30 minutes. Remove from refrigerator, slice into rounds and bake as above.

As a savoury pie base
Make the basic batter and press into pie dish. Bake as above. Cheese may be added as for cheese straws.

Sweet cookies
Add to the water and butter mixture:
2–3 level tablespoons sugar
1 teaspoon various flavouring essences (see below)
¼ teaspoon salt

Add any of the following to the cooled egg and almond mixture:

Plain biscuits
1 teaspoon vanilla essence

Almond biscuits
1 teaspoon almond essence

Chocolate chip cookies
1 teaspoon vanilla essence
125 g (4 oz) grated plain chocolate

Cherry cookies
1 teaspoon almond essence
125 g (4 oz) of chopped glacé cherries

Sultana or raisin cookies
1 teaspoon rum essence
125 g (4 oz) sultanas or raisins

Valencia cookies
1 teaspoon orange essence
50 g (2 oz) chopped orange peel

Sweet pie base
Make as for sweet cookies, but omit the flavouring essence. Press the mixture into the base of the prepared pie or cake tin. Add the filling and bake. For uncooked fillings the base must be cooked first.

Rich chocolate cake

Ingredients
250 g (9 oz) plain chocolate, not too bitter
175 g (6 oz) butter or margarine
75 g (3 oz) sugar or 25 g (1 oz) sugar and 2 tablespoons liquid honey
225 g (8 oz) ground almonds
1 teaspoon vanilla essence
4 eggs, separated
pinch salt
5 tablespoons apricot jam

Method
Line a 22 cm (8½ inch) round cake tin with baking parchment. Melt 175 g (6 oz) of the plain chocolate in a bowl set in a saucepan of simmering water. When melted, stand in a warm place.

Whisk the egg whites with a pinch of salt until stiff. Cream 125 g (4 oz) of the butter with the sugar and/or honey until light and fluffy. Add the egg yolks and continue beating until creamy. Stir in the melted chocolate, ground almonds, vanilla essence and blend well. Fold in the egg whites.

Pour into the tin and bake for 55–60 minutes in a moderate oven (160°C–180°C, 325°F–350°F, gas mark 3–4) or until done. Remove from oven and leave for a few minutes. Turn on to a wire rack and cool.

To ice the cake, warm the apricot jam slightly in a small saucepan over a low heat. Spread over the top of the cake and allow it to cool completely. Put the remaining chocolate and the butter in a bowl set into a saucepan of simmering water and melt together. Spread the apricot over the top of the cake, allowing the mixture to run down the sides. This cake may sink slightly when cooking, but any cracks in the surface will be covered by the apricot and chocolate topping.

Chocolate coffee cheesecake

Ingredients

1 rich chocolate cake (as opposite) without apricot and chocolate topping
1 tablespoon coffee liqueur (Tia Maria or Kahlua)
1 tablespoon milk
250 g (9 oz) unbranded cream cheese
75 g (3 oz) sugar
1 egg
3 teaspoons gelatine
2 tablespoons water
3 tablespoons coffee liqueur, extra
300 ml (10 fl oz) extra-thick cream
2 teaspoons cocoa
2 teaspoons starch-free icing sugar
75 g (3 oz) flaked almonds

Method

Slice the chocolate cake carefully into two rounds so that one layer is thicker than the other. Place the thicker layer on the bottom of a 22 cm (8½ inch) loose-bottomed cake tin which has been buttered and lined with baking parchment – a circle for the base and two strips around the side coming right up the tin. Reserve the other layer of cake for the top.

Brush the bottom layer with half the combined coffee liqueur and milk. Combine the cream cheese with the sugar and egg and beat until smooth.

Sprinkle gelatine over the 2 tablespoons of water in a small bowl. Set in a saucepan of simmering water and stir to dissolve. Add the extra coffee liqueur to the gelatine and blend with the cream cheese mixture. Blend in the cream. Pour the mixture into the cake tin over the cake base. Place the remaining layer of cake on top, brush with remaining coffee liqueur and milk mixture and refrigerate for several hours or overnight until set.

Remove from the tin. Peel the baking parchment away from sides and base, and place on a serving dish. Toast the flaked almonds by baking in a moderate oven for 5 minutes or until golden brown. Cool. Press the toasted almonds all over the cream cheese sides. Mix the cocoa and icing sugar together, put in a sieve and sprinkle over the top of the cake.

Amaretti biscuits (lactose-free)

Ingredients
125 g (4 oz) coarse ground almonds
175 g (6 oz) caster sugar
3 large eggs
1 teaspoon vanilla essence
1 teaspoon almond essence
½ teaspoon salt
blanched almonds for decorating

Method
Separate the egg whites, beat with the sugar and salt until stiff. Fold in ground almonds and essences. Place dessertspoonfuls on baking trays which have been covered with parchment and put one whole blanched almond on top of each. Bake in a slow to moderate oven (140°C–160°C, 290°F–325°F, gas mark 2–3) for 20–25 minutes, until lightly browned. Leave on the tray for a few minutes before removing to cool on a wire rack.

Amaretti wafers (lactose-free)

Method
Same recipe as above but put yolks in a separate bowl and beat last, until pale and thick. Fold almond mixture into yolks, blend well. Place on parchment and cook as above. Spreads thinner than biscuit recipe.

Florentines

Ingredients
125 g (4 oz) flaked almonds
25 g (1 oz) mixed peel
25 g (1 oz) glacé cherries – both red and dark if possible
1 tablespoon sultanas
12 g (½ oz) angelica
12 g (½ oz) glacé pineapple
4 good-quality dried apricots
75 g (3 oz) butter
3 tablespoons sugar or 1 tablespoon sugar and 2 tablespoons liquid honey
¼ teaspoon salt
1 tablespoon cream
125 g (4 oz) plain chocolate

Method

Finely chop the mixed peel, cherries, sultanas, angelica, pineapple and apricots. Melt the butter in a saucepan over a low heat. Add the sugar and salt. Stir until the sugar dissolves and bring to the boil. Boil gently for a minute without stirring. Just as mixture is beginning to turn a light brown, add the cream, fruit and nuts. Stir well.

Spoon the heaped teaspoonfuls on to well-greased oven trays, allowing plenty of room for spreading. It is best to bake only four at a time. Bake in a moderate oven (160°C, 325°F, gas mark 3) for about 10 minutes or until golden brown. Remove from the oven. Push each florentine into a neater round shape with a spatula. Allow to cool on the tray for one minute, then carefully lift each florentine from the tray on to a wire cooling rack. Cool completely.

Melt the chocolate in a bowl in a saucepan of simmering water. Allow it to cool slightly. Turn the biscuits over so that the flat side is uppermost. Spread a teaspoonful of chocolate on to each to cover. When almost cool, make wavy marks with a fork in the chocolate. Refrigerate until the chocolate is set. Store in an airtight container.

Meringues (lactose-free)

Ingredients

    3 egg whites
    150 g (5 oz) caster sugar
    ¼ teaspoon salt

Method

Prepare the baking tray by covering it with baking parchment. Beat the egg whites with salt until soft peaks form. Gradually beat in the sugar until stiff. Place small spoonfuls of meringue on a baking tray, or pipe from piping bag fitted with a plain piping tube approximately 2 cm (¾ inch) in diameter. Cook in a slow oven (130°C, 260°F, gas mark ½) for about an hour or until dry to the touch. Allow to cool with the oven door open. Remove from the parchment and stand on a cake rack. Store in an airtight container.

Almond and apricot meringue torte

Ingredients

4 egg whites
225 g (8 oz) caster sugar
¼ teaspoon salt
150 g (5 oz) chopped blanched almonds
80 g (just over 3 oz) dried apricots
1 tablespoon brandy
300 ml (½ pint) cream
350 g (12 oz) can of whole apricots

Praline

125 g (4 oz) sugar
2 tablespoons water
125 g (4 oz) chopped blanched almonds

Method

Place the almonds on an oven tray and bake in a moderate to slow oven for 5 minutes. Cool. Beat the egg whites with salt until soft peaks form. Add the sugar gradually, beating until completely dissolved. Fold in the first amount of almonds.

Butter two large oven trays, cover with baking parchment and butter again. Place half the meringue mixture on each tray in a matching round, about 25 cm (10 inches) diameter. Bake in a slow oven (130°C, 260°F, gas mark ½) for about an hour or until dry to the touch. Change the position of the trays halfway through baking time. Remove from the oven, remove from the baking parchment and cool.

Cover dried apricots with boiling water and allow to stand for 20–30 minutes. Drain and purée in a blender or processor. Stir in the brandy. Whip the cream until quite stiff and fold into the apricots. Spread one-third of the apricot cream over a meringue layer, top with the remaining layer, spread with the remaining cream, decorate with whole canned apricots and sprinkle with praline.

For the praline, place the sugar and water in a small pan, stir without boiling until sugar has dissolved, boil rapidly until a light golden colour, add the almonds, pour the mixture on to a lightly greased oven tray and allow to set. Break into pieces and chop finely in food processor.

Petite coffee meringues

A change from after-dinner mints.

Ingredients
1 egg white
¼ teaspoon salt
½ teaspoon white vinegar
75 g (3 oz) caster sugar
1 teaspoon starch-free icing sugar
2 tablespoons extra icing sugar
2 teaspoons instant coffee powder

Coffee cream
2 teaspoons instant coffee powder
1 tablespoon hot water
120 ml (4 fl oz) cream

Method
Sift all the icing sugar. Grease two oven trays and cover with baking parchment. Place the egg white, vinegar, salt and caster sugar in a small bowl and beat at high speed for about 10 minutes or until sugar is dissolved. Fold in 1 teaspoon of sifted icing sugar. Place teaspoonfuls on oven trays, trying to keep a uniform size, or pipe using a small plain piping tube. Bake in a slow oven (130°C, 260°F, gas mark ½) for about 40 minutes or until dry to the touch. Carefully remove from the baking parchment and cool.

For the coffee cream, dissolve the coffee powder in the hot water, cool and add to the cream. Beat until soft peaks form. Join meringues with the coffee cream, combine the remaining icing sugar and coffee powder and dust over the meringues on a serving plate.

Dawn's chocolate log

Because this cake contains no ground almonds, it is particularly delicate and may be difficult to remove, even from baking parchment. However, you should have no trouble if you butter the surface of a sponge roll tin or oven tray and cover with baking parchment, then butter the surface of the baking parchment.

Ingredients
3 eggs, separated
6 tablespoons caster sugar
75 g (3 oz) plain chocolate
1 tablespoon brewed coffee
about a tablespoon of sifted starch-free icing sugar
¼ teaspoon salt

Method
Melt the chocolate in a bowl over simmering water, add the coffee and cool. Beat the egg whites with salt until stiff. Beat the yolks with sugar until creamy. Add the chocolate and coffee mixture, beating to blend well. Gently fold in the stiff beaten egg whites.

With a rubber spatula, spread the mixture on to the prepared tin or tray in an oblong shape. Bake in a moderate oven (160°C–180°C, 325°F–350°F, gas mark 3–4) for about 15 minutes or until done. Remove from the oven and place a clean damp tea-towel over the cake. Turn upside-down on to the tea-towel, peel off the baking parchment and roll up along the length of the cake. Leave to cool. Unroll and fill with whipped cream. Reroll and dust with icing sugar.

Chocolate truffles

These have a hard, chewy consistency and a creamy taste because of the dried milk powder. They're full of calcium, so they're very good for you.

Ingredients
50 g (2 oz) butter
4 tablespoons caster sugar
4 tablespoons mild-flavoured honey
4 tablespoons milk
175 g (6 oz) plain chocolate
17 tablespoons dried milk powder – either low-fat or regular
vanilla essence
1 cup sultanas
ground almonds

Method
Measure the dried milk into a mixing bowl. In a saucepan over a low heat, melt the butter, milk, chocolate, sugar and honey together, add the vanilla and pour into the dried milk mixture. Add the fruit and stir well to blend. This mixture thickens as it cools and may become quite stiff. When blended, either roll into small balls and roll in ground almonds, or place in greaseproof paper or foil, roll into a log and slice to serve. Set in the refrigerator.

Chocolate raisin bars

Ingredients
50 g (2 oz) raisins
2 teaspoons brandy
1 small (170 g/6 oz) can Nestlé cream
75 g (3 oz) plain chocolate
125 g (4 oz) ground almonds
175 g (6 oz) milk chocolate or plain chocolate

Method
Sprinkle the brandy over the raisins and allow to stand for 2–3 hours. Place the first amount of dark chocolate in a bowl in a saucepan over simmering water and melt gently over a low heat. Add the cream and stir to blend. Remove from the heat, stir in the almonds and raisins and spread in an 18 cm x 18 cm (7 inch x 7 inch) buttered or non-stick baking

tin. Chill. Melt the remaining chocolate over simmering water and pour over the chilled base. Chill to set and cut into bars. Store in the refrigerator.

Raisin clafouti

Ingredients
>75 g (3 oz) raisins
>135 ml (4½ fl oz) milk
>350 g (12 oz) cottage cheese
>3 eggs
>75 g (3 oz) sugar
>¼ teaspoon salt
>50 g (2 oz) ground almonds
>50 g (2 oz) butter
>grated zest of 1 lemon
>1 tablespoon lemon juice
>starch-free icing sugar

Method
Line a rectangular oven-proof dish or loaf tin with baking parchment. Sprinkle the raisins over the bottom of the dish. Place the remaining ingredients in a bowl and blend until smooth. Pour over the raisins. Bake in a moderate oven (190°C, 375°F, gas mark 5) for 40–45 minutes or until the mixture is set and lightly browned. Remove and sprinkle with icing sugar. This can be served hot with cream as a pudding or cold as a cake.

Christmas cake

Ingredients
225 g (8 oz) butter
125 g (4 oz) white or brown sugar
4 tablespoons liquid honey
¼ teaspoon salt
6 eggs
350 g (12 oz) finely ground almonds
500 g (1 lb) seedless raisins
juice of 1 orange
225 g (8 oz) currants
225 g (8 oz) sultanas
125 g (4 oz) mixed peel
125 g (4 oz) chopped glacé cherries
grated zest of orange
85 ml (3 fl oz) brandy or sherry
1 teaspoon almond essence
1 teaspoon vanilla essence
1 teaspoon bicarbonate of soda

Method
Prepare a 20 cm (8 inch) square cake tin by lining it with two layers of brown paper and then with baking parchment. Wash the orange well, grate the zest and squeeze the juice. Cream the butter, sugar, salt and honey, and add the eggs one at a time. Mix in the grated orange zest, fruit, orange juice, brandy and essences. Mix the bicarbonate of soda with the ground almonds and add. You can add 2–3 more tablespoons of ground almonds at this stage if you think the mixture is too sloppy.

Pour into a cake tin and bake for 3½–4 hours in a very slow oven (120°C–140°C, 250°F–275°F, gas mark ½–1) or until a skewer or large darning needle comes out clean when inserted in the centre. Allow the cake to cool in the tin for several minutes, then remove from the tin and put on a wire rack. The cake can be iced with marzipan icing (make sure it is completely starch-free) topped with white icing made with starch-free icing sugar.

Rich chocolate cheesecake

Ingredients
   750 g (1½ lb) Mascarpone or ricotta cheese
   250 ml (8 fl oz) soured cream
   150 g (5 oz) sugar or 50 g (2 oz) sugar and 2 tablespoons liquid honey
   1 teaspoon vanilla essence
   3 eggs
   ¼ teaspoon salt
   225 g (8 oz) plain chocolate

Method
Prepare the cake tin as instructed in the 'Superb Cheesecake' recipe (see index). Melt the chocolate in a bowl over a saucepan of simmering water, then remove from the heat.

Beat the cheese with an electric beater until fluffy. Add the chocolate, soured cream, sugar/honey, vanilla and salt. Beat in the eggs one by one. Pour into the prepared tin and bake in a moderate oven (160°C, 325°F, gas mark 3) for 1 hour. If the cake springs back leaving no fingerprint when touched in the middle, it is ready. Turn off the oven and allow the cake to cool completely with the door opened. Refrigerate overnight. Serve with cream.

Easy Christmas pudding

This pudding can be steamed, but if you wish to boil it in the traditional way, have ready a 62-cm (25-inch) square of unbleached calico. Before using, drop it into a large pan of boiling water and boil for 30 minutes. Remove the cloth from the water and wring it out well. (You'll need rubber gloves!) Spread the cloth out and cover liberally with ground almonds. The cloth can be left uncoated, but this will give a better 'skin' on the pudding. Also have ready several yards of string (not twine!) and a very large saucepan three-quarters full of boiling water. There must be enough water for the pudding to float.

Ingredients
   1 kg (2 lb) mixed fruit, chopped if necessary
   3 eggs
   125 g (4 oz) white or brown sugar
   4 tablespoons liquid honey
   ¼ teaspoon salt
   250 ml (8 fl oz) cream
   85 ml (3 fl oz) brandy
   350 g (12 oz) finely ground almonds
   1 teaspoon bicarbonate of soda

Method

In a large basin, beat the eggs with the sugar, honey and salt until thick and creamy. Add the fruit, cream and brandy. Mix the bicarbonate of soda with the ground almonds and add to the fruit. Blend well. The consistency should not be too sloppy but this will vary depending on how finely the almonds have been ground. If you think it's necessary, add a few more tablespoons of ground almonds at this stage.

Turn out into the centre of the prepared cloth, gather the corners and sides around the pudding as evenly as possible, pull the corners tightly to give the pudding a good shape. Tie firmly with the string about 2.5 cm (an inch) or so from the top of the pudding mixture to allow room for expansion. Twist the string round the cloth about 10 times to give a good, firm seal. Make a handle from the string ends to lift the pudding out easily when cooked. Lower the pudding into water, put the saucepan lid on immediately and boil rapidly for 5 hours. Add more boiling water about every 20 minutes – the water must never go off the boil. When done, remove the pudding from pan and suspend it freely from the handle of a cupboard door or between the legs of an upturned stool or hook – the pudding must be able to swing freely without touching anything. Leave overnight. On the day of serving, reboil for a further 1½ hours. Serve with brandy butter or starch-free brandy sauce.

To steam, grease two 2-pint (1.2 litre) basins and pack the mixture into them. Cover each basin with a square of greaseproof paper and a square of pudding cloth on top. Secure them around the rim with string, or place the pudding basin lids over the greaseproof paper. Steam for 5 hours without letting the pudding basins touch the bottom of the pan or the water boil away. Cool and store. On day of serving, re-boil for 1½ hours.

Sauces and dressings

If you've only ever thought of sauces as being made with flour or cornflour, you're in for a pleasant surprise. Cream or wine sauces are delicious and very easy to make – cream *and* wine sauces are the ultimate. There really is never any need to thicken sauces with starch – they can all be made in other ways, whether we're talking about sweet or savoury sauces.

Standard crème fraîche sauce

This is a delicious substitute for any standard white sauce normally made with flour or cornflour. Many cooks wrongly think that crème fraîche will curdle if it is boiled – this is not so. The mixture will go through a curdling stage but if you continue boiling, it will reconstitute itself and become smooth.

Ingredients
250 ml (8 fl oz) crème fraîche
salt
juice of 1 lemon

Method
Place the crème fraîche over a gentle heat. Season to taste and simmer until thicker and smooth. Add the lemon juice and any of the following herbs or flavourings: chives, tarragon, chervil, marjoram or fish, poultry or meat juice. You can make it richer by adding a tablespoon of cream.

Mock béchamel sauce
Omit the lemon juice, add 25 g (1 oz) butter and a pinch of dried onion granules.

Mock mornay sauce
Make as for mock béchamel, but omit the onion granules. Remove from the heat and add half a cup (or so) of mild grated cheese (Emmental or Gruyère or other good melting cheese). Blend well and add two egg yolks, one at a time, beating hard with a wooden spoon. Return to a low heat and bring barely to simmering point. Remove and season to taste.

Hollandaise sauce

Here is a modern version of this classic sauce, made in a blender or food processor. If you want to make it the traditional way, you'll find the recipe in most books. Not all contain lemon juice but I prefer the flavour – you can omit it if you wish.

Ingredients   **Makes about 285 ml or 10 fl oz**
    2 egg yolks
    1½ tablespoons boiling water
    225 g (8 oz) butter
    1 tablespoon lemon juice
    salt to taste

Method
Gently melt the butter over a low heat without boiling. Skim the whey (white froth) off the top and pour the clear butter into a separate container, discarding any watery whey at the bottom of the original saucepan. Put the egg yolks in a blender or food processor, begin to blend on a low speed, slowly adding the boiling water and then the clear butter very slowly in a thin stream. Blend for a few seconds, add the lemon juice and a dash of salt. Check the seasonings. Serve quickly or keep warm over simmering water for no longer than an hour.

Mousseline sauce
Fold in 2 tablespoons of whipped cream.

Anchovy sauce (lactose-free)

Ingredients
    250 ml (8 fl oz) any starch-free mayonnaise
    1 clove garlic
    45 g (1½ oz) can anchovy fillets
    1 tablespoon starch-free tomato ketchup

Method
Drain and finely chop the anchovy fillets, crush the garlic and combine with the other ingredients.

Tartare sauce

Another modern easy-to-make version of a great classic.

Ingredients
   120 ml (4 fl oz) any starch-free mayonnaise
   1½ tablespoons soured cream
   2 teaspoons fresh dill
   1 teaspoon chopped chives
   2 teaspoons chopped parsley
   1 teaspoon capers rinsed in water to dilute brine
   3 spring onions
   1 teaspoon lemon juice
   salt to taste

Method
Combine mayonnaise, soured cream and lemon juice. Finely chop all the herbs and blend well. Taste before you add any extra salt.

No-starch gravy

Method
Roast the joint or poultry by itself using a recipe from this book or your usual method. Roast any potatoes and parsnips in separate dish, brushed with melted butter or olive oil and seasoned. To give the vegetables a better flavour, remove some of the roasting tin drippings from the meat during roasting and pour over vegetables.

Remove the joint to a serving dish and keep warm. Tilt the tin to allow the fat to rise to the surface and skim the fat from drippings. Replace the tin on a low heat. If you have cooked, say, a turkey or a joint of meat slowly over a long period, especially if it contains fruit stuffing, you may not need to add anything to the drippings to improve the flavour other than a cup of water or wine.

Instead of a stock cube
If the roasting tin drippings look pale and uninteresting you will want to add flavouring. Instead of a stock cube (which contains starch) you can now add any or all of these: a teaspoon of honey-mustard or any sort of French mustard that takes your fancy (as long as it contains no starch); a dash of lemon juice; 120 ml (4 fl oz) of red or white wine; a tablespoon of dried onions; a teaspoon of dried garlic; a pinch of herbs; a knob of butter. Stir all together over a slow heat, scraping the brownings from the bottom of the tin.

Instead of flour, gravy thickening or cornflour
Remove from the heat and add 1–2 tablespoons (depending on how brown you want the final mixture to be) of crème fraîche, Greek yoghurt or cream. Stir all together. Replace on the heat and slowly bring to the boil and allow the gravy to simmer until you have the desired consistency, adjusting seasonings and adding more wine or water if you wish. The consistency of the gravy may not be as thick as a flour-thickened sauce, but it will be more delicious and will thicken on standing.

Béarnaise sauce

Ingredients
  ½ teaspoon onion granules
  120 ml (4 fl oz) wine vinegar
  1 level tablespoon chopped tarragon
  2 tablespoons water
  salt
  2 egg yolks
  125 g (4 oz) butter

Method
Bring the vinegar to the boil, add the onion granules and simmer until the vinegar has almost completely evaporated. Meanwhile, chop the butter into knobs and set aside. Add the tarragon to the pan and remove it from the heat. Add the water and egg yolks, whisking vigorously with a wire whisk or electric beater until the mixture is frothy. Return the pan to a low heat, whisk in the butter, knob by knob. The sauce should now be thick and velvety.

Rich mustard sauce for steak

Ingredients
  50 g (2 oz) butter
  1 tablespoon brandy
  2 tablespoons red wine
  1 tablespoon coarse-grain French mustard
  120 ml (4 fl oz) cream

Method
Fry the steaks in butter or oil, or grill, as desired, remove and keep warm. Add the brandy to the pan drippings. Ignite the brandy, remove

the pan from the heat and allow the flame to die down. Stir in the mustard, wine and cream, then bring to the boil, stirring constantly until the sauce slightly thickens. Serve over the steaks.

Hot mustard sauce for gammon

Ingredients
1 *tablespoon Dijon mustard*
2 *tablespoons honey-mustard*
1 *tablespoon white wine vinegar*
1 *egg*
2 *tablespoons Greek yoghurt (or crème fraîche)*
120–250 *ml (4–8 fl oz) liquor gammon is boiled in*

Method
Whisk the mustards, egg and vinegar together in a saucepan. Slowly add half the liquor and whisk until blended over a low heat. Add the yoghurt or crème fraîche and continue stirring well until the mixture thickens. Add more liquor if needed and remove from the heat. Pour into a warm sauce boat. This sauce will continue to thicken on standing. Thin by adding more liquor.

Bitter orange sauce for game or pâté (lactose-free)

Ingredients
zest of 1 lemon
1 *tablespoon lemon juice*
1 *cup orange marmalade – preferably a bitter type*
2 *tablespoons sweet sherry or port*
1 *teaspoon honey-mustard*
4 *tablespoons water*

Method
Thinly peel the lemon with a potato peeler and cut the rind into thin strips about 5 cm (2 inches) long or use a zester. Bring the water to the boil in small saucepan and add the zest. Simmer for 5 minutes and remove from the heat. In another saucepan heat the marmalade over a slow heat until melted. Push through a sieve and discard the orange pieces. Return the marmalade to the pan, add the port or sherry and mustard. Squeeze the lemon juice and add to the marmalade with the water and lemon rind. Simmer gently over a low heat for a few minutes (leave the thin strips of zest in).

Garlic-cream sauce for fried chicken

Ingredients
½ teaspoon garlic granules
1 teaspoon honey-mustard or ½ teaspoon honey and ½ teaspoon Dijon mustard
1 tablespoon Greek yoghurt, crème fraîche or thick cream
50–120 ml (2–4 fl oz) wine or water
salt

Method
Fry the chicken as desired and remove to a warm plate. Pour away the surplus pan drippings leaving a couple of teaspoons in the pan. Add the wine or water (or both) and scrape down the pan brownings. Add the garlic granules and mustard and blend. Add the yoghurt or cream, blend well and allow to simmer for a few minutes. Season to taste. If you need to dilute it, add more wine or water.

Wine sauce for grilled steak (lactose-free)
Make in the same way as Garlic-Cream Sauce but do not use water and omit the yoghurt or cream. Red wine is best.

Fresh tomato sauce (lactose-free)

Can be frozen into ice-cube trays and stored in a plastic bag to be used as stock cubes. Measurements for this sauce are flexible. Sometimes I make more than at other times. Add more or less sugar/salt according to taste, and according to how sweet the tomatoes are. Can also be used as tomato soup, either hot or cold.

Ingredients
about 16 large plum tomatoes (you can use ordinary tomatoes but you may need to add more sugar)
4 or 5 large cloves of garlic, skinned, or 1 solo garlic
about 6 fresh bay leaves
2 teaspoons salt
2 tablespoons sugar
1–2 tablespoons olive oil

Method
Place the tomatoes in a bowl and pour boiling water over them to cover. Allow to stand until the skins are beginning to crack. Peel the garlic cloves and, if using solo garlic, peel and quarter. Put the oil in a large saucepan, add the garlic and gently simmer over a very low heat

until the garlic infuses the oil. Don't allow to brown. Remove from heat. Add the washed bay leaves. Take each of the tomatoes out of the hot water with a fork, slip the skins off and cut into quarters. Slice off the core. (Some people prefer to discard the seeds because they make the flavour less intense, but don't bother for this recipe as it is not intended to be a really intensely flavoured sauce.) This will be messy and lots of tomato juice will drip off. Have a colander ready to throw the skins and cores into.

Put the tomatoes into a food blender in batches, not adding too much at any time, and purée. If you add too much at a time the tomatoes at the bottom tend to get puréed while the ones at the top stay whole. Add the tomatoes to the saucepan as they are puréed. When they are all puréed, return the saucepan to the heat and slowly bring to the boil, stirring from time to time to stop browning. Add the sugar and salt. Taste and adjust seasonings. When it comes to the boil, remove from heat. Allow to cool completely and freeze.

This will keep in a glass jar in the refrigerator for a few days, if the top is covered with olive oil, but because it is not properly cooked it is better to store it frozen. My ice-cube trays produce a cube that is 2 x 2 x 1 inches, or 5 x 5 x 2.5 cms. Or freeze in plastic bags.

Tarragon sauce for grilled meats

Ingredients
175 g (6 oz) butter
2 level tablespoons Dijon whole-seed mustard
1 level tablespoon chopped tarragon

Method
Melt the butter in a small saucepan but do not let it brown. Add the mustard and tarragon. Stir well to blend, allow to heat through and serve.

Cheese and wine sauce for fish

Ingredients
50 g (2 oz) butter
125 g (4 oz) mild grated cheese such as Emmental or Gruyère
½ teaspoon garlic granules
1 tablespoon white wine
1 tablespoon cream
salt

Method
Melt the butter over a low heat in a saucepan, add the grated cheese, garlic and wine. Stir to blend well without browning on the bottom. Stir in the cream, and add salt to taste. The sauce can be thinned with more wine or milk. Serve hot over cooked fish or use as a cooking sauce when baking fish.

Sauce veronique

For grilled chicken or fish.

Ingredients
  250 ml (8 fl oz) dry white wine
  350 ml (12 fl oz) water
  65 ml (2½ fl oz) dry vermouth
  50 g (2 oz) butter
  120 ml (4 fl oz) cream
  125 g (4 oz) white seedless grapes

Method
Combine the wine, water and vermouth in a medium-sized saucepan. Boil rapidly until it is reduced by half. Reduce the heat, add the butter and cream and stir until thickened. Add the grapes, reheat without boiling and serve.

Fresh tarragon sauce

For grilled meats, chicken or fish.

Ingredients
  50 g (2 oz) butter
  ½ teaspoon garlic granules
  2 tablespoons fresh tarragon
  1 teaspoon mild Dijon mustard
  1 teaspoon lemon juice
  65 ml (2½ fl oz) brandy
  120 ml (4 fl oz) cream

Method
Heat the butter, garlic, tarragon, mustard, lemon juice and brandy until boiling. Reduce heat and simmer uncovered for 2 minutes. Gradually stir in the cream, reheat without boiling, and serve.

Best vinaigrette (lactose-free)

Because I eat salad almost every day, I make up this vinaigrette in bulk in a blender and store in a 1 litre extra-virgin olive oil glass bottle.

Ingredients   **Makes 1 litre (1¾ pints)**
 2 teaspoons best rock or sea salt
 7 teaspoons sugar
 ¾ cup any mixed vinegars, or you could use just one type
 3 cups extra-virgin olive oil

Method
In a bowl, stir the salt and sugar with the vinegar until dissolved. Measure oil into blender. Add dissolved mixture. Blend. Pour into storage bottle. This mixture will separate on standing but does not need to be stored in refrigerator, unless you wish. Shake the bottle well and pour a small amount into a separate bottle or container to serve.

Mint sauce (lactose-free)

Ingredients
 3–4 handfuls fresh mint leaves
 2 tablespoons granulated sugar
 120 ml (4 fl oz) light malt vinegar
 boiling water
 salt to taste

Method
Place the mint leaves on a large chopping board and chop coarsely with a large, sharp knife. Sprinkle with the sugar and chop finely, holding the handle of the knife in one hand and the tip in the other. As the sugar and leaves become scattered, scrape them into a small pile and continue chopping, until the leaves are very fine and well incorporated into the sugar. Scrape into a small bowl or jug, barely cover with a little boiling water then add the vinegar and salt to taste. More sugar or vinegar can be added if desired.

Classic vinaigrette (lactose-free)

Ingredients
> 1 tablespoon wine vinegar
> 2½–3 tablespoons best olive oil
> 1 clove garlic
> salt

Method

Peel the garlic, chop roughly on a chopping board, sprinkle with salt and crush with the blade of a knife, scraping up, sprinkling more salt and crushing again until a paste. Measure the vinegar and olive oil into a jar, add the garlic and shake until blended.

Make your own variations by adding any of these: a teaspoon of Dijon mustard; a pinch of sugar; ½ teaspoon of honey; any non-starch seasonings such as steak seasoning, Italian garlic seasoning, etc. You should test them for starch before using. Aromatic vinegars, fruit vinegars, malt vinegars or lemon juice can also be substituted for wine vinegar.

Slimmer's salad dressings

Version one ingredients
> ½ teaspoon garlic granules
> 1 teaspoon Dijon mustard – any sort
> 150 ml (5 oz) mild unflavoured low-fat yoghurt
> 1 tablespoon lemon juice
> ½ teaspoon non-starch tomato ketchup

Method

Combine all the ingredients and blend well. Store in the refrigerator.

Version two ingredients
> 1 tablespoon low-fat yoghurt
> 1 tablespoon Greek full-fat yoghurt
> 1 teaspoon honey-mustard
> salt and pepper to taste

Method

Combine all ingredients and blend well. Store in the refrigerator.

Caesar salad dressing

Ingredients
   50 g (2 oz) grated Parmesan cheese
   175 ml (6 fl oz) lemon juice
   250 ml (8 fl oz) light olive oil
   120 ml (4 fl oz) extra-virgin olive oil
   50–80 g (2–3 oz) can anchovies
   1 teaspoon strong Dijon mustard
   2 cloves fresh garlic, peeled
   2 hard-boiled eggs

Method
Put all the ingredients in a food blender and blend well.

Honey lime dressing (lactose-free)

Ingredients
   250 ml (8 fl oz) vegetable oil
   120 ml (4 fl oz) lime juice
   120 ml (4 fl oz) honey
   1 tablespoon grated lime zest
   ½ teaspoon celery seed

Method
Wash the lime well, grate and squeeze the juice. Combine with the
other ingredients.

Yellow Brick Bank dressing (lactose-free)

A genuine recipe from the Wild West, named after an old bank.

Ingredients
   500 ml (18 fl oz) olive oil
   120 ml (4 fl oz) red wine vinegar
   1 egg
   2 cloves garlic, peeled and crushed
   2 teaspoons sweet Dijon mustard
   ½ teaspoon dried oregano
   ½ teaspoon dried dill
   salt

Method
Combine all the ingredients in a blender. Store in the refrigerator.

Creamy blue-cheese dressing

Ingredients
>   70 g (about 2½ oz) blue cheese
>   120 ml (4 fl oz) cream
>   3 tablespoons lemon juice
>   ½ teaspoon fresh or dried chervil
>   1 teaspoon fresh or dried tarragon
>   pinch garlic granules
>   salt to taste

Method
Mash the blue cheese in a bowl, add the cream slowly and blend well – or blend in food processor. Add the remaining ingredients and blend again.

Green goddess salad dressing

Ingredients
>   120 ml (4 fl oz) starch-free mayonnaise
>   85 ml (3 fl oz) soured cream
>   1 tablespoon tarragon vinegar
>   1 tablespoon lemon juice
>   ½ teaspoon dried onion granules
>   2 anchovy fillets
>   1 tablespoon chopped chives
>   2 tablespoons chopped parsley
>   1 clove garlic, crushed

Method
Blend all the ingredients in an electric blender or food processor. Serve cold.

Old-fashioned orange sauce

Ingredients
  25 g (1 oz) sugar
  1 tablespoon grated orange zest
  120 ml (4 fl oz) fresh orange juice
  50 g (2 oz) butter
  3 large eggs, lightly beaten
  1 tablespoon lemon juice
  pinch salt

Method
Combine all the ingredients in the top of a double boiler, or in a bowl inserted into a saucepan a quarter filled with water (do not let bowl touch bottom of saucepan). Stir well. Bring the water to the boil, reduce the heat so that the water is just simmering. Cook, stirring constantly, until the mixture is smooth and thickened. Serve warm or cold over ice-cream or cheesecake.

Apricot sauces

Version one ingredients
  325 g (12 oz) can sugar-free apricots
  2–3 tablespoons sugar
  25 g (1 oz) butter
  1 tablespoon apricot brandy (optional)

Method
Blend the apricots until smooth in a blender or push through a sieve. Place in a saucepan with the sugar and butter and bring to the boil. Simmer for a few minutes, remove from the heat and add the apricot brandy. Serve warm.

Version two ingredients (lactose-free)
  175 g (6 oz) dried apricots
  500 ml (18 fl oz) water
  125 g (4 oz) sugar
  1 tablespoon rum (optional)

Method
If the dried apricots are very hard, chop finely and soak overnight in the water. Add the sugar, then bring the chopped fruit to the boil,

reduce heat, simmer for 15 minutes or so until the apricots are tender. Cool. Sieve or blend with the syrup in which they have been cooked until smooth. Add the rum.

Melba sauce (lactose-free)

Ingredients
> 1 pack (approx 350 g) frozen raspberries
> 4 tablespoons sugar
> 1 jar good blackberry jelly (jam), such as Tiptree

Method
Defrost the raspberries and purée in a food processor. Push through a fine sieve to remove the seeds. Place in a saucepan with the sugar and bring to the boil. Simmer for a few minutes, remove from the heat and add the blackberry jelly, stirring until well blended. If the jelly does not melt into the hot raspberries, return to the heat for a few minutes, but try to combine them without extra cooking. Refrigerate and serve chilled.

Hot fudge sauce

Version one ingredients
> 250 g (9 oz) sugar
> 175 g (6 oz) butter
> 125 g (4 oz) plain chocolate
> 2 tablespoons milk
> dash salt

Method
Grate the chocolate into the sugar in a saucepan. Add the milk, stir well and place over a low heat. Add the butter, melt together and bring slowly to the boil. Taste and add salt. Boil for about 3 minutes, stirring constantly. Remove from the heat. This is a very rich sauce – less butter can be added if desired. Do not overcook as it will become too hard when cool.

Version two ingredients
> 75 g (3 oz) plain chocolate
> 250 ml (8 fl oz) soured cream
> 125 g (4 oz) sugar and 120 ml (4 fl oz) mild-flavoured honey
> 1 teaspoon vanilla essence

Method
Combine all the ingredients in the top of a double boiler or a bowl set into a saucepan of simmering water. Cook, stirring occasionally, for about an hour. This sauce will be thick and will keep for several weeks in the refrigerator. Makes about 500 ml (18 fl oz).

Caramel sauce

Ingredients
225 g (8 oz) sugar
75 g (3 oz) butter
400 ml (14 fl oz) cream
dash salt

Method
Place the sugar, butter and half the cream in a saucepan. Bring to the boil over a low heat, stirring frequently. Boil for a few minutes then stir in the remaining cream. Taste and add salt. Boil for a minute or so extra, remove from the heat and serve warm.

Brandy sauce for Christmas pudding

Ingredients
2 tablespoons sugar
120 ml (4 fl oz) water
2 egg yolks
pinch salt
2 tablespoons brandy
120 ml (4 fl oz) cream, whipped

Method
Place the sugar and water in a saucepan over a low heat and stir until the sugar dissolves. Bring to the boil, reduce the heat and simmer for 10 minutes. Beat the egg yolks and salt. Remove the hot sugar syrup from the heat and pour slowly into the eggs, beating until thick and creamy. Fold in the brandy and cream.

Sweets

The most reliable way to test the cooking of sweets is with a sugar thermometer. But I have never had one. Instead, I learned the hard way – beginning at the age of about eight or nine, making toffee and fudge with my brothers and sisters, and never getting it right until we mastered the trick of the 'ball-in-the-water' test. It was a lot of fun, involving many tastes. We each had our own cup of cold water and usually consumed so much of the stuff in various soft and hard ball stages that we were utterly sick of it when it was finally ready.

Here's how to test it. When it has been cooking for about the right amount of time as specified in the recipe, drop a little into a cup of cold water. Wait a few seconds and then test it between your fingers. If the right temperature has been reached, it will roll into a little ball, and depending on what you're making, this is how the balls should feel:

Fudge or caramel – a soft ball – not runny or sloppy but a definitely formed, soft ball that holds its shape.

Toffee and butterscotch – a hard ball – it should chink when you knock it against the side of the cup. This will produce a hard but chewy toffee. Some recipes say it should 'snap'. This means that the moment you pour it into the cold water it will immediately harden and become very brittle. This will be very hard toffee.

Toffee (lactose-free)

Ingredients
> 225 g (8 oz) sugar
> 120 ml (4 fl oz) water
> 2 tablespoons vinegar
> ¼ teaspoon salt

Method
Place all the ingredients in a heavy saucepan over a medium heat. Stir until the sugar dissolves, then boil, unstirring for 15 minutes or to a hard-ball stage. Pour into a buttered dish and cool. Mark into squares before it is completely hard.

Chocolate fudge

Ingredients

120 ml (4 fl oz) milk (evaporated milk gives a lovely creamy flavour)
50 g (2 oz) plain chocolate, grated
500 g (1 lb) sugar
125 g (4 oz) butter
1 teaspoon vanilla essence
¼ teaspoon salt

Method

Mix the sugar, salt and chocolate together in a saucepan. Add half the butter and slowly heat, stirring until the chocolate is blended in. Add the milk, stirring. Bring to the boil, stirring occasionally, then boil until the soft-ball stage. Remove from the heat. Cool for 5 minutes. Add the rest of the butter and vanilla. Beat until thick, then pour into a buttered dish before it sets. Mark into squares and cut before completely hard.

Butterscotch

Ingredients

125 g (4 oz) butter
120 ml (4 fl oz) cold water
500 g (1 lb) sugar
1 teaspoon cream of tartar
pinch salt

Method

Put the butter, sugar, salt and water into a saucepan. Heat slowly and when the butter is melted, add the cream of tartar and boil for about 15 minutes or until the very-hard-ball stage. Pour into a buttered dish and allow to cool. Mark into squares and cut before completely hard.

Cream caramels

Ingredients

675 g (1½ lb) sugar
125 g (4 oz) butter
475 ml (16 fl oz) cream
½ teaspoon salt

Method

Bring the sugar, butter, salt and half of the cream to the boil, stirring constantly. Add the rest of the cream and continue boiling, stirring frequently until the hard-ball stage. Pour into a buttered dish and cut into squares when cold.

Toffee apples

Ingredients

 725 g (1½ lb) sugar
 1 tablespoon vinegar
 1 tablespoon butter
 4 tablespoons cold water
 ½ teaspoon cream of tartar
 drop of red food colouring

Method

Have a number of apples ready on toffee apple sticks. Boil all the ingredients together in a heavy-based saucepan without stirring until the very-hard-ball stage. Remove from the heat, dip the apples into the liquid toffee, then stand upside-down on baking parchment until hard.

Truffles

Ingredients

 50 g (2 oz) butter
 75 g (3 oz) plain cooking chocolate
 175 g (6 oz) icing sugar
 1 tablespoon rum
 chocolate sprinkles

Method

Heat the butter and chocolate in a saucepan over a moderate heat until melted. Remove from the heat, add half the icing sugar and stir until thick. Add the rum and enough icing sugar to make a stiff mixture. Shape into small balls and roll in the chocolate sprinkles.

Relishes

I have not yet come across a commercially made chutney or relish that could be eaten on a non-starch diet. Most contain cornflour or other starch thickening. Fruit jelly or jam is a very good substitute to eat with cold meats or cheese. Redcurrant and cranberry jelly are traditional with game and ham, but if the general idea horrifies you, it is simply because you may not realise how similar 'jam' is to the chutneys and relishes with which you are familiar. They're both cooked in the same way with sugar – chutneys and relishes usually include vegetables, but not always; jams and jellies are sometimes made with vegetables, such as tomatoes and marrows. The main difference is that the chutneys and relishes have the distinctive flavour of vinegar and spices. You can achieve a very good substitute for this by combining jelly and mustard made with vinegar, such as Dijon mustard or honey-mustard.

Mustard fruits (lactose-free)

Ingredients
1 pear
1 apple
1 orange
50 g (2 oz) green grapes
50 g (2 oz) black grapes
425 g (14½ oz) can black cherries
1½ tablespoons mixed peel
10 cloves
350 ml (12 fl oz) red wine vinegar
350 ml (12 fl oz) water
350 g (12 oz) sugar
2 tablespoons hot Dijon mustard

Method
Sterilise two large preserving jars by immersing them in cold water with their lids and caps, bring to the boil and boil for 15 minutes. Leave the jars in the water until needed. Remove them one at a time.

Peel and core the pear and apples, cut into eighths, then cut each slice in half. Wash and dry the grapes, drain the cherries. Place the fruit in a large bowl, add the mixed peels and cloves and toss gently.

Meanwhile place the wine vinegar, water and sugar in a saucepan, stir over a medium heat until the sugar dissolves, bring to the boil, reduce the heat and boil gently for 5 minutes. Pack the fruit into the hot, sterilised jars. Add the mustard to the vinegar mixture, stir until combined. Stand the jars of fruit in a bowl or sink so that it doesn't matter if they overflow and pour the vinegar mixture over the fruit in the jars to cover completely. Keep for a week before opening and refrigerate when opened. Makes about 1 litre (2 pints).

Plum-orange chutney

This is quite tart, almost a sour mixture – a good substitute for piccalilli.

Ingredients (lactose-free)
   24 large plums
   1 large orange
   850 g (1¾ lb) seedless raisins
   120 ml (4 fl oz) cold water
   120 ml (4 fl oz) honey
   2–3 tablespoons hot Dijon mustard

Method
Wash the plums well, pat them dry, remove the stones and cut into chunks. Wash the orange well and pat dry. Peel the zest thinly with a potato peeler, taking care not to include the bitter white pith, or use a zester. Remove all the pith and dice the pulp small. Cut the zest into very small pieces. Place the plums, orange pulp and zest, raisins, honey and water in a saucepan, bring to the boil and cook over a medium heat, stirring frequently until thick (about 45 minutes). Remove from the heat, stir in the mustard (taste and add more if you wish). Pour into sterilised jars as described in Mustard Fruits.

Plum sauce (lactose-free)

Use instead of tomato sauce.

Ingredients
   1.5 kg (3 lb) plums
   900 ml (1½ pints) malt vinegar
   400 g (14 oz) sugar
   2 teaspoons whole cloves
   1–2 tablespoons honey-mustard

Method
Wash the plums well and remove the stones. Put all the ingredients except the honey-mustard into a large saucepan and boil together until reduced to a pulp (about 2½–3 hours). Remove from the heat, then stir in the honey-mustard to taste. Push through a sieve or blend until smooth. Pour into sterilised jars as described in Mustard Fruits.

Prunes in red wine (lactose-free)

Ingredients
> 250 g (9 oz) pitted prunes
> ½ bottle red wine
> sprig of thyme
> sprig of rosemary
> 1 bay leaf
> strip of lemon rind
> 1 tablespoon sugar
> 1 teaspoon honey-mustard

Method
Combine the wine, herbs, lemon rind and sugar in a saucepan and boil until the liquid is reduced by about a half. Strain and return to the saucepan. Add the prunes and cook gently until plump and tender (10–15 minutes), remove from the heat and stir in the honey-mustard. Pour into sterilised jars with the liquid. Store in a cool place.

Orange curd

Ingredients
> juice of 3 large oranges
> 3 eggs
> 75 g (3 oz) butter
> 225 g (8 oz) sugar

Method
Whisk the eggs, sugar and juice together in a small bowl until blended. Place the bowl over a saucepan of simmering water (or in the top of double boiler), add the butter and cook, stirring, until thick. Cook for a further 15 minutes. Pour into sterilised jars.

Flavoured butters

These are wonderful as toppings for grilled or fried steaks, chicken or fish. Combine the ingredients in a food processor, or with an electric mixer. Turn out on to greaseproof paper or foil, roll into a log shape and freeze until needed. Slice on to hot food.

Herb butter

125 g (4 oz) lightly salted butter
2 tablespoons lemon juice
1 teaspoon chopped fresh thyme
2 teaspoons chopped fresh watercress
½ teaspoon chopped fresh rosemary
1 tablespoon chopped fresh parlsey

Roquefort butter

125 g (4 oz) lightly salted butter
90 g (3½ oz) Roquefort cheese
1 teaspoon grated lemon zest
1 teaspoon hot Dijon mustard

Maître d'hôtel butter

125 g (4 oz) lightly salted butter
2 teaspoons lemon juice
2 tablespoons chopped parsley
1 tablespoon chopped fresh chives

Stuffings

Fruit stuffing for turkey

This gives enough stuffing for a small turkey of about 3.5 kg (6½ lb) – probably about half the size of most people's Christmas turkey. Increase the recipe for a larger bird.

Ingredients
150 g (5 oz) stoned soft eating prunes
250 g (9 oz) soft dried apricots
300 g (10 oz) (about 3 medium-sized) eating apples
3 tablespoons dried mixed herbs – any sort
1 tablespoon garlic Italian seasoning (optional)
¼ teaspoon onion salt
¼ teaspoon onion granules
1 teaspoon garlic granules
sprinkle of salt
2 eggs

Method
Chop the dried fruit finely and place in a large mixing bowl. Peel and grate the apples, pouring away any excess juice and add to the dried fruit. Add all the seasonings and mix. Add the two eggs and mix again to blend all the ingredients. At this stage the stuffing may look too sloppy – don't worry as the eggs will bind it during the cooking.

Remove the turkey from its packaging and untruss. Remove giblets, etc., from neck- and leg-end cavities. Push stuffing into both ends of the bird, folding down the flap of skin at the neck end to hold the stuffing in, and pinning the leg end with cocktail sticks. Cook the turkey as desired.

New apple-less turkey stuffing (lactose-free)

Because I am having increasing trouble getting starch-free apples, I prefer to use this stuffing. The amount of starch in sweet apples may not affect everyone, but if you want to play safe, this is a delicious stuffing. You will notice that as opposed to the fruit stuffing with apples, this one contains about twice as much prunes as apricots. This is because without apples, the sharpness of the apricot flavour tends to dominate. Instead of apples I now add tomatoes, which may sound a strange combination with the dried fruit, but it actually tastes really good. The amounts are fairly flexible. Don't worry if you don't have exactly the right measurements, and increase measurements as required for a larger turkey. This stuffing keeps the turkey deliciously moist.

Ingredients   **To stuff a 3.5 kg (6½ lb) turkey**

250 g (9 oz) soft eating prunes
150 g (5 oz) soft dried apricots
500 g (1 lb) (about 4 largish) bland tomatoes
250 g (9 oz) smoky bacon, either streaky or back
3 tablespoons dried mixed herbs, any sort
1 teaspoon onion granules (optional)
1 teaspoon garlic granules (optional)
1 egg
125 g (4 oz) dairy-free spread

Method
Dice the bacon. Chop the fruit and the tomatoes. Put all in a basin and add herbs and granules. Mix all into a sludgy mass with the dairy-free spread. Beat the egg with a fork just to blend it and mix into the other ingredients. Don't worry if it looks too sloppy. It will all hold together after cooking. Remove the turkey from its packaging, untruss, remove giblets, etc., from neck and leg-end cavities. Push stuffing into both ends of the bird, folding down the flap of skin at the neck end to hold the stuffing in and either sewing or pinning the leg end with cocktail sticks. Follow cooking instructions for roast turkey (see index).

Drinks (lactose-free)

All these drinks contain fruit sugar (fructose) and are ideal to serve at a party, because fructose increases the rate of alcohol metabolism and can help prevent hangovers. You can use fruit sugar as a replacement for ordinary sugar in your favourite punch or squash recipes. It's worth going to a little extra trouble to get fruit sugar for drinks because it increases the fruit flavour. But if you can't, use caster sugar.

Peach sangria

Ingredients   **Serves four**
   750 ml (1¼ pints) Chablis or other dry white wine
   4 tablespoons peach schnapps or brandy
   3 tablespoons fruit sugar
   1 fresh peach, peeled and thinly sliced
   1 orange, thinly sliced
   1 lemon, thinly sliced

Method
Combine the first three ingredients in a large jug, stirring until the sugar is dissolved. Add the fruit, cover and chill for at least an hour. Strain and pour into a serving jug. Serve over ice, adding fruit to each glass.

Amazing fruit squash

Ingredients
   350 ml (12 fl oz) bottle or pack of orange or pineapple juice
   175 g (6 oz) fruit sugar
   1 teaspoon citric or tartaric acid

Method
Mix all the ingredients together and make up to 2.25 litres (4 pints) with water. More sugar or honey can be added to taste.

Strawberry champagne punch

Ingredients

3 punnets strawberries
125 g (4 oz) fruit sugar (more to taste)
85 ml (3 fl oz) Grand Marnier
2 tablespoons lemon juice
1.5 litres (2½ pints) (2 bottles) champagne

Method

Wash and hull the strawberries and allow to dry. Save half a punnet and place the rest of the strawberries in a blender or processor, add the sugar, Grand Marnier and lemon juice, blend on high speed until puréed. Place the strawberry mixture in punch bowl. Just before serving add the cold champagne and remaining chopped strawberries. Make about 2.5 litres (4½ pints).

Handy hints

Make your own stock 'cubes' (lactose-free)

Save any roasting tin drippings from roast meat or poultry. Pour into a container and allow to settle. Refrigerate. The meat juices will set into a jellied stock underneath the fat. When needed, skim the fat off the top and add the jellied juice to gravies, soups or any savoury dishes. The stock from chicken cooked with lemon juice and herbs makes an especially nice addition to salad dressings. If the fat is well skimmed off before cold, the meat juices can be poured into ice-cube trays and frozen into cubes.

Herb cubes

Chop washed and dried fresh herbs, either in single varieties or mixed, and pack into ice-cube trays, adding a little water to hold in place. Freeze. Store the frozen cubes in freezer bags and use as required, simply adding to the dish during preparation.

Fresh herbs
Can also be frozen unblanched. Separate the washed and dried leaves from the stalks and store in small freezer bags. Chop or crumble into food while still frozen.

Snacks

Marinated olives (lactose-free)

Ingredients
2 cans pitted Spanish olives
about 1 tablespoon raspberry or red wine vinegar
about 3 tablespoons extra-virgin olive oil
generous sprinkle dried herbs
several large cloves garlic, skinned

Method
Drain olives and combine all ingredients. Store covered in fridge. Eat as snack or use as ingredient for other recipes.

Salted almonds (lactose-free)

Do use good rock or sea salt – it makes a huge difference. These taste wonderful warm, and even better chilled.

Ingredients
600 g (1¼ lb) blanched whole almonds
garlic-infused olive oil or plain olive oil (does not need to be extra-virgin)
rock salt

Method
Into a heavy-bottomed frying pan (stainless steel if possible) over a low heat, pour enough oil to cover pan. Add enough almonds to cover the bottom. Roast slowly, shaking the pan from time to time. Toss after a few minutes until a golden-brown colour. Don't over-roast. Have ready a dish lightly covered in coarsely ground rock salt. Spoon the roasted almonds on to this and grind more rock salt over the top. Continue roasting another batch, until all are cooked, salting each layer. If you oversalt, wait until cool, put them all in a colander and shake until the surplus salt is shaken off. Store in the refrigerator in a covered jar. Long storage time.

Espresso ice-cream

Out and about in the big city, feeling down and out – what can I eat? Here's something you can get in most restaurants, snack bars and coffee bars. First time I saw someone order this, I was impressed. It seemed the height of casual chic and tastes great too and will quickly boost your energy levels.

Ingredients
    2 scoops vanilla ice-cream
    1 espresso (small, strong cup of coffee)

Method
Pour coffee over ice-cream and eat.

Silly snacks

Other people will think you're silly, but it tastes great! You need a packet of best-quality eating dates – the sort you buy for Christmas – some unbranded cream cheese (not Philadelphia) or some lightly salted butter (I prefer the butter). Slit each date open, remove the stone, place a sliver of cream cheese or butter inside date and eat. Great when you need something sweet. Similar to date scones – without the scone!

Savoury snacks

Thin slices of good Cheddar cheese wrapped in lettuce leaves make a quick and easy substitute for a sandwich.

Blue cheese is wonderful with sweet apples.

Cream cheese and chives are great with celery.

Try some thin processed cheese (or Dutch breakfast cheese) wrapped around a slice of ham or salami spread thinly with redcurrant jelly.

Try a slice of starch-free pâté on a slice of tomato.

Sophisticated snacks

Wash one or two small sweet apples, quarter them, remove the cores and cut into about eight slices. Cook in hot butter for about 3–4 minutes, turning once. Place on lettuce leaves on a plate and crumble some farmhouse Cheshire or crumbly Cheddar cheese over, add a squeeze of lemon juice and eat.

Sordid snacks

Pure greed and the secret knowledge that leftover baked apples may look awful but they taste great invented this snack. Scrape the cooked, chilled flesh away from the skin, mash with a fork and fold into an equal amount of plain mild yoghurt or whipped cream.

REFERENCES

America's Best Recipes, Oxmoore House, Inc., 1993.

Australian Family Circle, *Cheesecakes, Puddings and Pies*, Advertiser Magazines Pty Ltd.

The Australian Women's Weekly, *Best Ever Recipes*, Australian Consolidated Press.

——, *Best Recipes from the Weekly*, Australian Consolidated Press.

——, *Best Ever Slimmers' Recipes*, Australian Consolidated Press.

——, *The Best Seafood Recipes*, Australian Consolidated Press.

——, *French Cooking Made Easy*, Australian Consolidated Press.

——, *Italian Cooking Class Cookbook*, Australian Consolidated Press.

'Bulley Fare', The Volunteers of Theodore Roosevelt Inaugural National Historic Site, 1991.

Bailey, Adrian, *DK Pocket Encyclopedia, Cook's Ingredients*, Dorling Kindersley Ltd, 1991.

Barasi, Mary E. and Mottram, R. F., *Human Nutrition*, Edward Arnold, 1992.

Beeton, Mrs, *Book of Household Management*, Ward Lock and Co, 1906.

Belle Entertaining, Australian Consolidated Press, December/February 1990.

Better Homes and Gardens New Cook Book, USA, 1961.

Booth, Christopher C. and Neale, Graham, *Disorders of the Small Intestine*, Blackwell Scientific Publications, 1985.

Braley, James and Hoggan, Ron, *Dangerous Grains*, Avery, 2002.

Calin, Andrei and Taurog, Joel D. (ed.), *The Spondylarthritides*, Oxford University Press, 1998.

Cannon, Geoffrey, *Superbug, nature's revenge*, Virgin Publishing Ltd, 1995.

Claire, Marie, *Cuisine Extraordinaire*, Conran Octopus, 1988.

Clark, Charles, *The New High Protein Diet*, Vermilion, 2002.

Colden Country Cookbook, Colden United Methodist Women, New York, 1990.

Concise Family Medical Handbook, Collins, 1986.

Concise Medical Dictionary, Oxford University Press, 1987.

Crocker, Betty, *Betty Crocker's Picture Cook Book*, USA, 1959.

Currie, Donald J., *Abdominal Pain*, Hemisphere Publishing Corporation, 1979.

David, Elizabeth, *French Country Cooking*, Penguin Books, 1966.

Davies, Dr Stephen and Stewart, Dr Alan, *Nutritional Medicine*, Pan Books, 1987.

Davis, Adelle, *Let's Eat Right to Keep Fit*, Unwin Paperbacks, 1979.

——, *Let's Get Well*, Unwin Paperbacks, 1979.

Dear, K. L. E. and Hunter, J. O., 'Irritable bowel syndrome, Crohn's disease and ulcerative colitis', in *Food Allergy and Intolerance*, ed. J. Brostoff and Stephen J. Challacombe, Saunders, 2002.

Dwyer, John M., *The Body at War*, Allen & Unwin, 1989.

Eades, Michael R. and Eades, Mary Dan, *Protein Power*, Thorsons, 2000.

Ebringer, Alan, 'Ankylosing Spondylitis is caused by *klebsiella*', *Spondyloarthropathies*, Rheumatic Disease Clinics of North America, Volume 18, number 1, February 1992.

—— and Wilson, C., 'The Use of a Low Starch Diet in the Treatment of Patients Suffering from Ankylosing Spondylitis', *Clinical rheumatology*, 1996, 15, suppl. 1.

—— and ——, 'Ankylosing spondylitis and diet', in *Food Allergy and Intolerance*, eds. J. Brostoff and Stephen J. Challacombe, Saunders, 2002.

——, Rashid, T. and Wilson, C., *Ankylosing Spondylitis as an Autoimmune Disease Caused by Intestinal Klebsiella Infection: Prospects for a New Therapeutic Approach*, Trustees of the Middlesex Hospital, the Arthritis Research Campaign (Grant EO514) and 'American Friends of King's College London'.

——, Bains, M., Childerstone, M., Ghuloom, M. and Ptaszynska, T., 'Etiopathogenisis of Ankylosing Spondylitis and the Cross-Tolerance Hypothesis', in *Advances in Inflammation Research, Vol. 9: The Spondyloarthropathies*, ed. M. Ziff and S. B. Cohen, Raven Press, 1985.

Edmonds' Cookery Book, Edmonds Food Industries Ltd, 1986.

Ensminger, Audrey H., Ensminger, M.E., Konlande, James E. and Robson, John R.K., *Concise Encyclopedia of Foods & Nutrition*, CRC Press, 1995.

Farmer, Fannie Merritt, *The Fannie Farmer Cookbook*, Bantam Books, 1983.

Fox, Brian A. and Cameron, Allan G., *Food Science, Nutrition and Health*, Edward Arnold, 1992.

Freed, David L.J., 'Dietary lectins and disease', in *Food Allergy and Intolerance*, eds. J. Brostoff and Stephen J. Challacombe, Saunders, 2002.

Galvani, Patrick, *Safeway Fresh Food Cookbook*, Octopus Books Ltd, 1984.

Goddard, Liza and Baldwin, Ann, *Not Naughty But Nice*, Ward Lock Ltd, 1987.

The Good Cook: Fish and Shellfish, Time Life Books, 1981.

Grieve, Mrs M., *A Modern Herbal*, Penguin Books, 1984.

Griffith, H. Winter, *The Complete Guide to Symptoms, Illness & Surgery*, Diamond Books, 1997.

Hanssen, Maurice, *E for Additives: The Complete E Number Guide*, Thorsons Publishers Ltd, 1987.

Hunter, J.O., 'Infections of the gastrointestinal tract and food intolerance', in *Food Allergy and Intolerance*, eds. J. Brostoff and Stephen J. Challacombe, Saunders, 2002.

Johnson, Leonard R. (ed), *Gastrointestinal Physiology*, The C.V. Mosby Company, 1981.

Khan, Muhammad Asim, *Ankylosing Spondylitis, the facts*, Oxford University Press, 2002.

Loes, M., Wikholm, G., Shields, M. and Steinman, D., *Arthritis: The Doctors' Cure*, Keats Publishing, Inc., 1998.

McCance and Widdowson, *The Composition of Foods*, Royal Society of Chemistry, fifth revised and extended edition, 1992.

McElroy, Mark and Sadler, John, *GCSE Chemistry*, Longman Revise Guides, Longman, 1988.

McFarlane, Shona, *White Moas and Artichokes: Paintings, Prose and Preserves*, Hazard Press, 1993.

Neale, Graham, *Clinical Nutrition*, Heinemann Medical Student Reviews, Heinemann, London.

NZ Truth Cookery Book, Wellington.

1000 Cooks' Hints, Treasure Press, 1991.

Parish, Peter, *Medicines: A Guide for Everybody*, Penguin Books, 1987.

Patten, Marguerite, *Cookery in Colour*, Hamlyn Publishing Group Ltd.

Read, N. W. (ed), *Gastrointestinal Motility, Which Test?*, Wrightson Biomedical Publishing Ltd, 1989.

Roden, Claudia, *Mediterranean Cookery*, BBC Books, 1987.

Sears, Barry, *The Zone*, ReganBooks, 1995.

Slater, Nigel, *Real Fast Food*, Penguin Books, 1992.

Slimming: The Complete Guide by the Experts of Slimming Magazine, Collins, 1993.

Smith, Anthony, *The Body* (revised edition), Viking, 1986.

Smith, Mike, *Dr Mike Smith's Postbag, Arthritis*, Kyle Cathie Limited, 1996.

Souli, Sofia, *222 Recipes: The Greek Cookery Book*, Michalis Toumbis Publications SA, 1989.

Stewart, Maryon and Stewart, Dr Alan, *The Vitality Diet*, Optima, 1992.

Tarr, Yvonne Young, *The Ten Minute Gourmet Cookbook*, Lyle Stuart Inc, 1965.

365 Savoury Suggestions (second edition revised), Whitcombe & Tombs Ltd.

Venes, Donald (ed.), *Taber's Cyclopedic Medical Dictionary*, F. A. Davis Company, 1997.

Vogue Australia Entertaining Guide Winter '93, Bernard Leser Publications Pty Ltd, 1993.

——, *Wine and Food Cookbook*, Bernard Leser Publications Pty Ltd, 1989.

Waddell, Gordon, *The Back Pain Revolution*, Churchill Livingstone, 1998.

Weighley, Emma S., Mueller, Donna H. and Robinson, Corinne H., *Robinson's Basic Nutrition and Diet Therapy*, Prentice-Hall, Inc., 1997.

Woman's Day, *Step by Step Cookbook*, Magazine Promotions Australia Pty Ltd, 1984.

Workman, Elizabeth, Alun Jones, Dr Virginia, Hunter, Dr John, *The Food Intolerance Diet Book*, Optima, 1986.

FEEDBACK

If you have found this book a help I would love to hear from you.

Over the last few years I have received many letters from people who have found the low-starch diet literally life changing. Some were suffering from irritable bowel syndrome (IBS), some had been diagnosed with the arthritic condition of ankylosing spondylitis (AS). But for some, it was the first time they had received any information that their many, various symptoms – including IBS, joint and back pain – were all symptoms of a real disease, and not just all in the mind. We are planning to feature some of you on our website as a means of helping others overcome their particular problem.

You can email us at: lowstarchdiet@attglobal.net

Or you can visit the website: www.lowstarchdiet.net

PERMISSIONS

The author and publisher are grateful for kind permission from Elsevier Science, Ltd., to publish edited quotations in chapter 5, from pages 1 and 2 of *The Back Pain Revolution*, by Gordon Waddell; and in chapter 11, edited quotations from pages 479, 482 and 484 of *Food Allergy and Intolerance*, edited by Jonathan Brostoff and Stephen Challacombe, chapter 34, *Dietary lectins and disease*, by David L. J. Freed.

Permission has also kindly been granted by Oxford University Press to publish an edited quotation in chapter 5, from pages 251 and 252 of *The Spondylarthritides*, edited by Andrei Calin and Joel D. Taurog, chapter 17, *'The Patient's Point of View'*, by Fergus J. Rogers.

Permission has also kindly been granted by Macmillan Publishers Ltd., to publish an edited quotation in chapter 13, from pages 302 and 303 of *Nutritional Medicine* by Dr Stephen Davies & Dr Alan Stewart.

INDEX